Risky Genes

Ashkenazi Jews have the highest known population risk of carrying specific mutations in the breast cancer genes BRCA1 and BRCA2. So what does it mean to be told you have an increased risk of genetic breast cancer because you are of Ashkenazi Jewish origin? In a time of ever-increasing knowledge about variations in genetic disease risk among different populations, there is a pressing need for research regarding the implications of such information for members of high-risk populations.

Risky Genes provides first-hand intimate descriptions of women's experiences of being Jewish and of being at increased risk of genetic breast cancer. It explores the impact this knowledge has on their identity and understanding of belonging to a collective. Using qualitative data from high-risk Ashkenazi women in the UK, this book elucidates the importance of biological discourses in forging Jewish self-identity and reveals the complex ways in which biological and social understandings of Jewish belonging intersect.

In *Risky Genes*, Jessica Mozersky reflects upon and offers new insight into the ongoing debates regarding the implications of genetic research for populations, and of new genetic knowledge for individual and collective identity. The book will be of interest to students and scholars of sociology, anthropology, Jewish studies, medical genetics, medical ethics, religious studies, and race and ethnic studies.

Jessica Mozersky is a Postdoctoral Researcher at the University of Pennsylvania's Center for the Integration of Genetic Healthcare Technologies (Penn CIGHT). She received her PhD in Anthropology from the interdisciplinary Institute of Human Genetics and Health at University College London. In 2011 she was selected to be a Visiting Researcher at the Brocher Foundation in Hermance, Switzerland. She is a founding member of an international comparative social science BRCA network, and has managed international multi-centre clinical trials for BRCA carriers and women at increased genetic risk of breast and ovarian cancer at University College London and King's College London.

Genetics and Society

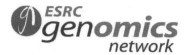

Series Editors: Ruth Chadwick, *Director of Cesagen, Cardiff University*, John Dupré, *Director of Egenis, Exeter University*, David Wield, *Director of Innogen, Edinburgh University* and Steve Yearley, *Director of the Genomics Forum, Edinburgh University.*

The books in this series, all based on original research, explore the social, economic and ethical consequences of the new genetic sciences. The series is based in the Cesagen, one of the centres forming the ESRC's Genomics Network (EGN), the largest UK investment in social-science research on the implications of these innovations. With a mix of research monographs, edited collections, textbooks and a major new handbook, the series is a valuable contribution to the social analysis of developing and emergent biotechnologies.

Series titles include:

Risky Genes

Genetics, breast cancer and Jewish identity

Jessica Mozersky

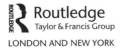

Routledge
Taylor & Francis Group

LONDON AND NEW YORK

First published 2013
by Routledge
2 Park Square, Milton Park, Abingdon, Oxfordshire OX14 4RN

Simultaneously published in the USA and Canada
by Routledge
711 Third Avenue, New York, NY 10017

First issued in paperback 2014

Routledge is an imprint of the Taylor & Francis Group, an informa business

British Library Cataloguing in Publication Data
A catalogue record for this book is available from the British Library

Library of Congress Cataloging-in-Publication Data
Mozersky, Jessica.
Risky genes: genetics, breast cancer and Jewish identity / Jessica Mozersky.
p. cm. – (Genetics and society)
Includes bibliographical references and index.
1. Breast–Cancer–Risk factors. 2. Cancer–Risk factors. 3. Jewish women–
Health risk assessment. 4. Women–Health risk assessment. I. Title.
RC280.B8M69 2013
616.99′449071–dc23
2012006198

ISBN 13: 978-0-415-50228-3 (hbk)
ISBN 13: 978-1-138-82284-9 (pbk)

Typeset in Times New Roman
by Taylor & Francis Books

Contents

Preface

The research carried out for this book, as is often the case, was born out of both personal and professional experience. On a personal level, I am a Canadian-born Ashkenazi Jewish woman without a family history of breast cancer who was raised in a secular family. Despite this secular upbringing, I belong to a generation of North American Jews whose parents, while often being liberal and even atheist, still felt a need to instil a 'Jewish' upbringing in their children. This could take the form of Hebrew school on weekends, bar or bat mitzvahs, trips to Israel, celebrating the major Jewish holidays and many other things as well. In my case it meant attending a Jewish day school until the age of 13, where I learned Hebrew, studied Jewish history and was surrounded by only Jewish classmates. I grew up believing that being Jewish was a religious/ethnic/cultural identity and not a biological one. The history of the Holocaust was something I learned about at Jewish day school and although I was never formally taught this, I knew very early on that the notion that Jews are a race or biological group was problematic, and even racist.

In 2002 I began to work in the UK on clinical research specifically for women at high genetic risk of breast and ovarian cancer. This professional experience was my first introduction to the high-risk breast cancer genes – BRCA1 and BRCA2 – and more importantly to the increased risk of genetic breast cancer for Ashkenazi Jews. I had never heard of the BRCA genes before then, nor of the importance and prevalence of Ashkenazi Jews in medical genetic research and discourse more generally. I was surprised and felt slightly ill at ease. Why were clinicians and scientists (Jewish or not) talking so often about Ashkenazi Jews and their diseases and genetic predispositions? Wasn't this reminiscent of some prior historical time when Jews were thought of as separate and biologically inferior?

My thoughts were further confounded by discussions I had with colleagues, including those from the biological sciences, and one particular conversation I had in 2004 stands out in my memory. This was the first time I was seriously confronted with the notion that being Jewish could also be considered biological because one had to be born into it. Most Jews were not a result of conversion but of being born to Jewish mothers who had long practised endogamy. My colleagues kindly explained to me that the history of endogamy among Jews had biological consequences and one way in which this was manifested was in the increased incidence of certain genetic diseases. I was uncomfortable, intrigued and fascinated by this. It entirely made sense and was consistent with my understanding that one needed to be 'born Jewish' (ideally to a Jewish mother) and with my familiarity with Tay-Sachs disease. Yet it simultaneously conflicted with my personal discomfort at talking about Jews as a biological group.

Of course, there are no answers to these questions and this book reveals that there is no such thing as a 'social' or 'biological' identity, and that Jewish identity very often comprises both in surprising and contradictory ways. However, throughout this research I have questioned my own understanding of what 'being Jewish' means and this complexity of identity is reflected in the ways in which individuals described and talked about being Jewish to me.

Acknowledgements

First and foremost I would like to thank the women, and men, who shared their stories with me, granting me a glimpse into their lives.

I owe a very large debt of gratitude to Professor Barbara Prainsack, who not only suggested that I pursue publishing this material as a book, but has also encouraged and supported me since the first time we met. I have also received tremendous support from Professor Dame Hazel Genn and Professor Nanneke Redclift, who guided me throughout the process.

I would also like to thank the anonymous reviewers whose comments, insights and suggestions helped me to refine and hopefully improve the book. Helen Greenslade, editorial manager at the EGN BOOK series, has provided excellent advice and support. Fintan Power's copy-editing skills are much appreciated.

This research was funded by the Institute of Human Genetics and Health at University College London. The questions, ongoing debate and exposure to different disciplinary standpoints that I received from my colleagues at this institute were invaluable to broadening my perspective and allowed me to have a more critical eye for all disciplines.

My first experience of working in the field of breast cancer genetics came via the Cancer Research UK and UCL Cancer Trials Centre, which stimulated my ongoing interest in this area. The centre was also extremely flexible with my employment there throughout this research.

Writing this book was made possible by a stay at the Fondation Brocher in Hermance, Switzerland (www.brocher.ch). I was incredibly fortunate to spend six months there as a visiting researcher, where the beautiful environment and stimulation of other researchers allowed me to complete this book. Special thanks to Dena Davis, Bob Cook-Deegan, Reed Pyeritz and Alison Cool for reading and/or discussing various aspects of the book with me (occasionally aided by a glass of wine), and to all the wonderful and caring staff at the foundation who made my stay unforgettable.

The Center for the Integration of Genetic Healthcare Technologies (CIGHT) at the University of Pennsylvania has also generously supported me during the final stages of this book.

Thanks to all of my friends and family, especially my parents Joy and Dan, and to Lolly and Josh, for their enduring support as I made my way through.

Last, but by no means least, thanks to my beloved Rob for his infinite patience, kindness, love and, above all else, humour.

Large portions of the following papers are reprinted in this book with permission from the publishers: Mozersky, J. (2012) 'Who's to blame? Accounts of genetic responsibility and blame among Ashkenazi Jewish women at risk of BRCA breast cancer', *Sociology of Health and Illness*, June, 34 (5): 776–90, Blackwell Publishing; Mozersky, J. (2011) 'Repensando las consecuencias de las investigaciones de genetica medica en las poblaciones: el caso de los judios Ashkenazi' (Rethinking the consequences of genetic research for populations: the case of Ashkenazi Jews), *Perspectivas Bioéticas*, 16 (30): 101–22, Facultad Lationoamericana de Ciencias Socialies; Mozersky, J. and Joseph, G. (2010) 'Case studies in the co-production of populations and genetics: the making of "at risk" populations in BRCA genetics', *Biosocieties*, 5 (4): 415–39, Palgrave Macmillan.

Introduction

I'm always really happy when I meet someone Jewish … it's hard to explain …
I am not particularly Jewish but it's a recognition …
        (Sarah, late forties, breast cancer survivor, no BRCA mutation found)

I think that you know the rabbis in their pulpits should be telling the women
actually … there's got to be more awareness amongst the women themselves
'cuz if they knew that there was an increased risk then they could take steps to
do something positive and constructive to help themselves really …
        (Jennifer, early forties, family history, awaiting genetics appointment)

The identification of the high-risk breast cancer genes – BRCA1 and BRCA2 –
in 1994 and 1995 respectively was accompanied by much hope and anticipation
both in terms of improving the diagnosis and treatment of breast cancer and also
more broadly regarding the potential of knowledge arising from the human
genome project. The *New York Times* described the 'massive hunt' for the breast
cancer genes as the greatest genetic enterprise since Gregor Mendel began
crossing his peas (Angier 1994). Shortly thereafter, it was also discovered that
Ashkenazi Jews (those of Eastern European descent) have the highest known
population risk of carrying three specific mutations in the BRCA genes, commonly referred to as the 'Ashkenazi BRCA mutations' (Antoniou et al. 2000,
Levy-Lahad et al. 1997). Ashkenazi Jews have an estimated 1 in 40 risk of
carrying BRCA mutations compared to a general population risk of between 1
in 400 and 1 in 800. Mutations in the BRCA genes confer a significantly increased
lifetime risk of developing breast cancer, up to 85 per cent, and although they are
most widely associated with breast cancer, they also confer a 10–40 per cent
increased risk of ovarian cancer (Antoniou et al. 2003). The discovery of the first
Ashkenazi mutation was announced in a press release in 1995:

This finding offers the first evidence from a large study that an alteration
in the gene, called breast cancer 1 (BRCA1), is present at measurable
levels not only in families at high risk for the disease, but in a specific
group of the general population.
        (National Cancer Institute 1995)

This new knowledge about Ashkenazi Jews' increased risk of genetic breast cancer was in some ways unsurprising. First, this information reflected the increasing interest in population, or racial and ethnic, differences in health and disease as a result of the human genome project. Second, Ashkenazi Jews have long been subjects of genetic research and much is known about genetic diseases in this population. Genetic breast cancer is the most recent addition to the substantial list of genetic diseases which Ashkenazi Jews have an increased risk of suffering. Screening programmes and research centres for 'Ashkenazi Jewish genetic diseases' exist throughout the world. Ashkenazi Jews are the most well researched in relation to genetic disease, are over-represented in human genetics literature and have historically been actively involved in research and genetic screening programmes (Birenbaum Carmeli 2004).[1] This has led to claims that Ashkenazi Jews are particularly supportive of genetic research and medicine related to them, and they are often considered to be the exemplar of a population that advocates and participates in research and screening programmes (Kronn et al. 1998, Lehman et al. 2002, Levin 2003, Rapp 2000).

The involvement of Ashkenazi Jews both as subjects and advocates of medical genetic research is a complex and somewhat paradoxical story. On the one hand, genetic and biological thinking about the difference or inferiority of Ashkenazi Jews has historically been used to justify anti-Semitism (Gilman 1985, 2003, Glenn and Sokoloff 2010). The eugenics movement of the early twentieth century and the Holocaust are stark reminders of the terrible consequences that have resulted from biological thinking about group difference for Ashkenazi Jews and many other populations. On the other hand, despite this history of discrimination, Ashkenazi Jews have been involved in medical genetic research especially in the post-war period, and with remarkably varied consequences. Today much is known about genetic diseases that occur at increased incidence among Ashkenazi Jews, screening programmes exist throughout the world, and the incidence of many diseases has been reduced as a result. Yet, the involvement and over-representation of Ashkenazi Jews have also been double-edged and illustrate both the benefits and drawbacks of genetic research for populations.

This book is an effort to explore and understand this somewhat paradoxical relationship, and in particular the consequences of genetic disease knowledge for individual and collective Jewish identity. This research contributes to two broader debates. The first concerns the utility of populations within genetic research and the potential implications for the populations being researched. The consequences are generally assumed to be negative and include increased discrimination, stigmatization or misunderstanding about the biological basis of racial or ethnic group differences. The major criticisms of research focused on Ashkenazi Jews are based on past misuses, especially during the Second World War, or potential future misuses of genetics (Gilman 2003, 2006) and are usually not based on empirical data. Amidst the controversy regarding populations and genetics, this research examines how Ashkenazi Jews have come to be so well represented in research and whether individuals have concerns about research focused on Ashkenazi Jews. If they are supportive, what might the reasons for this be? The second area of debate relates to the potential of new genetic knowledge to transform individual and collective identity and alter how individuals conceive of themselves and the groups to which they belong. This book explores the implications for individuals of knowing that they are at increased risk of genetic breast cancer because they are of Ashkenazi Jewish origin. It specifically addresses whether being at increased risk has an impact on how such women feel about their own Jewish identity and understanding of belonging to a collective. In exploring these questions, the co-production (Jasanoff 2004) of science and society and the 'social' nature of genetic medicine will be revealed.

Before turning to these two particular debates, and in order to contextualize them, it is first necessary to turn our lens backwards and briefly examine the long and contentious history of the scientific classification of racial or ethnic groups.

Historical context

Biological theories of racial difference have existed for many centuries and the word 'race' first became widely used in Europe in the sixteenth and seventeenth centuries (Bamshad et al. 2004, Obasogie 2009). These theories proposed that there were inherent biological differences between races, although how race was defined has been variable and included continental, national and religious groups (Obasogie 2009). Early categorizations corresponded to continental divisions and are often still used today. In the nineteenth century, a more systematic attempt to categorize racial groups began and science played a key role in understanding race at this time (Obasogie 2009). Early biological theories of race assumed there was an unchangeable biological basis to race and class, and racial and class stratification were therefore justified because differences were rooted in biology. Rose (2007: 160) refers to the use of genetics and biology to justify social inequality and discrimination as 'biogenetic legitimation'. Physical, mental, moral and behavioural characteristics were all believed to be hereditary, and theories proposed biological evolution and the superiority of particular races, usually White Europeans and Americans. Biological explanations were used to legitimate many of the social inequities and prejudices of nineteenth-century Europe, including to justify colonialism, discrimination and slavery (Gould 1981). Francis Galton, the English anthropologist and father of eugenics, defined eugenics as 'giving the more suitable races or strains of blood a better chance of prevailing speedily over the less suitable' (Galton 1883: 17). Biological arguments led to eugenic programmes of forced sterilization, whereby those who were deemed to be biologically inferior, including the poor, criminal and mentally ill, were forcibly sterilized (see Cowan 2008). At its worst, such biological thinking about 'racial' differences provided the underlying justification for the Nazi persecution of the Jews. The

Holocaust saw the mass murder by the Nazis of six million Jews who were deemed to be biologically inferior, and this remains a significant aspect of Jewish history for many Jews throughout the world (Zertal 2000). Nazi ideology sought to justify the genocide of Jews by likening Jews to a 'cancerous lesion' that 'sullied the "pure" body of the German body' (Clow 2001: 296). Other groups, including Africans, homosexuals and the mentally ill, were also systematically murdered by the Nazis.

Following the Second World War, and in direct response to the Nazi atrocities that had occurred, there was an overwhelming shift in thinking about race (Fujimura et al. 2008, Marshall 1993, Obasogie 2009, Skinner 2007). In 1950 UNESCO issued the following statement:

> The biological fact of race and the myth of 'race' should be distinguished. For all practical social purposes, 'race' is not so much a biological phenomenon as a social myth [which has] created an enormous amount of human social damage.
>
> (UNESCO 1950: 8)

While this statement does not deny that there may be biological differences between races, it explicitly acknowledges the severe harm that resulted from such thinking about group differences. This statement also clearly separates 'biological' and 'social' concepts of race. The second half of the twentieth century was dominated by thinking about race as a social construct (Skinner 2007). The social construction theory of race is used to convey the idea that the importance placed on outward physical distinctions that societies have used to draw racial boundaries varies over time and place, that these physical distinctions do not reflect any inherent meanings, abilities or disabilities, and that racial differences in social or health outcomes do not correlate meaningfully with underlying biological or genetic mechanisms (Obasogie 2009: 3). Many scholars view race as a sociohistorical construct and have argued that racial categories should be studied as political, social and cultural, as opposed to biological, categories (Fujimura et al. 2008, Marshall 1993, Obasogie 2009, Skinner 2007). Shared ethnic culture, origin myths, religion or nationality can all be the basis upon which individuals are distinguished as a race and these do not necessarily have a biological basis (Skinner 2007: 936). For example, in Brazil over 40 racial categories exist and siblings can be from different races (Marshall 1993).

While the frequency of biological discussions about racial differences declined (although they never ceased) following the Second World War, they resurfaced after the publication of the first draft of the Human Genome Project. One of the most acclaimed findings following the first draft publication in 2000 was that humans were 99.9 per cent genetically alike.[2] This figure was used to support the idea that racial differences were social rather than genetic, and many social and scientific researchers viewed this as potentially moving society beyond biological thinking about race (Obasogie 2009: 2). US

President Bill Clinton made the following statement after the first draft of the human genome project was completed:

> I believe one of the great truths to emerge from this triumphant expedition inside the human genome is that, in genetic terms, all human beings, regardless of race, are more than 99.9 per cent the same. What this means is that modern science has confirmed what we first learned from ancient fates. The most important fact of life on this Earth is our common humanity.
>
> (White House, Office of the Press Secretary, 26 June 2000)

Despite this, there was an immediate interest in the 0.1 per cent difference, which researchers argued could translate into biomedically significant variability (Fujimura et al. 2008). Research into genetic variation between populations has focused on two main areas – medical genetics and population genetics. Medical research looks for genetic variation in disease and drug response among populations, while population research examines what genetic variation can tell us about the migration and ancestral history of various populations. Research projects in both these areas proliferate.[3] One large and well-known project is the HapMap Project. HapMap is an international collaboration to find genetic similarities and differences between African, Asian and European populations that affect health, disease and drug response. They are using samples from the Yoruba in Nigeria to represent African ancestry, Han Chinese in Beijing and Japanese in Tokyo to represent Asian ancestry and from Utah residents to represent Northern and Western European ancestry. Currently the 1000 Genomes project is using whole genome sequencing on 1,000 individuals derived from more diverse groups including East Asians, West Africans, the Americas and Europe to provide a more comprehensive resource on human genetic variation.[4]

A note about terminology

Within the scientific and non-scientific literature, the terms race, ethnicity and population are all used in varying contexts with slightly different, yet often overlapping, meanings. Throughout the twentieth century race has had no standard definition in medical, epidemiological or health services research, and there are no agreed upon definitions for the terms race and ethnicity (Braun et al. 2007, Collins 2004, Ellison et al. 2007). Genetic articles sometimes use the terms race and ethnicity as though they are synonymous (Bradby 1996), and Ellison et al. (2007) found that scientists often adopted the term 'ethnicity' in preference to 'race' because they believed it was more socially acceptable. Risch et al. (2002) acknowledge that race and ethnicity are often used interchangeably by geneticists, and they define racial groups as those based on the primary continent of origin, whereas ethnicity is a 'self defined construct that may be based on geographic, social, cultural, and religious grounds' (Risch et al. 2002: 3). They claim that ethnicity can have potential meaning from a genetic perspective if it defines endogamous groups that can be 'differentiated from other such groups' (Risch et al. 2002: 3). Within scientific literature, the term population is most commonly used to refer to groups that are genetically differentiated from one another because of historical, geographical and/or cultural separation. However, the population categories used in medical research cross a variety of boundaries that may include geography, ancestry, 'race', religion and nationality and represent groups ranging from the highly endogamous to the highly admixed (admixture refers to reproduction across groups). Significant difficulties remain when it comes to defining what constitutes a population due to the permeability and porous boundaries of populations. Chapter one contains a further discussion of how and why Ashkenazi Jews are considered a population from a genetic standpoint. Throughout this book I have used the term population in an attempt to avoid some of the baggage that terms such as race and ethnicity carry, and because it is the dominant term used in medical genetics. However, I recognize that this term is itself problematic and there is a huge amount of overlap between groups however they may be defined.

It is also worth stating at the outset that there is no single unified group of Ashkenazi Jews, and this research is not an attempt to be representative of 'Ashkenazi Jews' or 'Jewish' identity or views as a whole. This is neither desirable nor possible given the tremendous diversity of Ashkenazi Jews and the lack of any single unified or easily identifiable 'community'. Jewish views are not a monolithic whole and this qualitative ethnographic research provides a window into the experiences of a particular sample of Ashkenazi Jews living in London, England.

In the following section I return to the two relevant debates for this book – the implications of genetic research and knowledge for identity and for populations.

Genetics and population

While the use of populations, or racial and ethnic groups, is a central strategy in medical genetics for attempting to understand human disease, it remains a highly contested area in both scientific and social scientific communities (Bamshad et al. 2004, Bradby 1996, Brodwin 2002, Duster 1990, 2006, Epstein 2007, Foster and Sharp 2002, Fujimura et al. 2008, Fullwiley 2007, 2008, Gilman 1985, 2003, 2006, Marks 2008, Risch et al. 2002). It has been claimed that searching for genetic variations, especially in relation to health and disease, could lead to an over-emphasis on the role of genetics as the basis for health disparities. Social determinants of health may take a back seat despite the fact that studies continue to reveal that poverty, environment, lack of education and other social determinants are more relevant to health disparities than genetics (Caulfield et al. 2009, Fujimura et al. 2008, Montoya 2007, Obasogie 2009, Ossorio and Duster 2005). Biological claims about health differences between groups could influence the ways in which social disparities are understood and lead to biological notions of racial difference (Caulfield et al. 2009, Montoya 2007, Obasogie 2009). This could allow old theories of racial minorities' supposed biological inferiority to be legitimated in new and different terms (Obasogie 2009: 14). Duster (2005: 1050) warns against the 'fallacy of reification'; the very use of these categories in genetics and medicine has the potential to render them real. Research projects that search for racial differences in disease susceptibility could 'reinscribe race through genetic technologies or produce genetic categories of race' (Fujimura et al. 2008: 647). Montoya (2007: 95) claims that ethnoracial categories are ill-defined biomedical constructs but it is crucial to distinguish between the two modes in which they are used – descriptive and attributive. As a descriptive tool, ethnoracial categories are used in scientific publications to report which human group specific biological samples and data were derived from. However, the labels can also be used to attribute qualities to groups and this can modify and delimit the groups being referred to, leading to racialization of groups.

It has also been claimed that research could lead to discrimination and stigmatization of those groups who become irrevocably linked with disease (Caulfield et al. 2009). Scientists are aware of the potential ethical issues that may arise; the HapMap project acknowledges that such research could

> raise risks of group stigmatization or discrimination, if a higher frequency of a disease-associated variant were found in a population and the risks associated with that variant were over generalized to all or most of the members of the population. Another potential concern is that the inclusion of populations based on ancestral geography could result in categories such as 'race', which are largely socially constructed, being incorrectly viewed as precise and highly meaningful biological constructs.
>
> (HapMap Project 2011)

Scientists are also aware of the deficiencies in using race, especially self-identified race, as a proxy for underlying genetic variation, and there is a substantial amount of literature and discussion regarding the relevance or not of race in genetic research, much of it from within the scientific community itself. There is disagreement regarding whether race actually corresponds to meaningful genetic variation, and while most geneticists deny a simplistic notion of race as a biological category and there remains no consensus on its definition or utility, the use of such categories in research continues nevertheless. Some argue strongly in favour of the importance of race and ethnicity in determining susceptibility to disease and drug response that could be useful in terms of diagnosis and treatment (Risch et al. 2002). In contrast, others, including the world renowned population geneticist David Goldstein, claim that race is only an interim solution to carry us through a 'period of ignorance' about the underlying causal factors of disease (Tate and Goldstein 2004: S39). For the most part the discussion is much more complex and the existence or relevance of race can be neither entirely dismissed nor justified by geneticists (see Bamshad et al. 2004). This led Francis Collins (2004: S14) to claim 'one could conclude that both points are correct'. Montoya (2007: 101) accurately points out that 'debates about race and ethnicity cannot be reduced to a race–no race binary position'.

The specific concerns about genetic research of the Ashkenazi Jewish population focus on potential continuities with historical misuses of genetics and anti-Semitism, and the possibility of Jews being labelled as more ill and facing discrimination or stigmatization as a result. Historically Jews in Europe have been associated with a propensity for ill health and disease, and this was often part of other anti-Semitic campaigns or beliefs about the inferiority of the Jews (Gilman 1985, 2003). Gilman (2003) warns that current genetic findings may lead to a return to the past or result in renewed discrimination and stigmatization, or an increase in racism towards Jews. This is a problem not only for Jews, but for any group that has historically been labelled as diseased or is currently associated with genetic illness. For Gilman, the past is reason enough not to pursue current genetic research. These criticisms, as well as how individuals felt about genetic research, are the subject of chapter three.

The concerns about the implications of genetic research for populations have two commonalities. First, they tend to rely on the past and historical abuses as a result of genetics to warn about concerns for the future. Second, the majority of criticisms tend to describe populations who are disempowered or disadvantaged, which may not always be the case. While there are of course many groups who are disadvantaged socio-economically, politically (and in many more ways), and there are ample historical examples of the misuse of genetics (see Duster 1990, Gilman 1985, Reardon 2005, Wailoo and Pemberton 2006), these two themes dominate discussions of genetics and population in general. The trajectory of Ashkenazi Jews within genetic medicine has been very different from that of some other populations such as African Americans, where the history of sickle cell screening or Tuskegee experiments in the United States have contributed to an overall distrust of the medical system and lack of participation, and representation, in genetic medicine (Duster 1990, Wailoo and Pemberton 2006).

While it is not my intention to oversimplify the critiques of many of those who raise concerns about genetic research and population, or to imply that such critiques always assume the consequences will be negative, I want to take a different approach and direct attention to the fact that there is a tendency to focus almost exclusively on the potential harmful consequences, while simultaneously not including the voices of members of the populations being described themselves.[5] In this book, empirical qualitative data on high-risk Ashkenazi Jewish women in the UK is used to examine the ways in which knowledge of being at increased risk of genetic disease is interpreted and experienced by members of a 'high-risk' population. This analysis does not therefore rely on history only, although this is a topic which inevitably arises. A drawback of this approach (or rather what is *not* examined) is that it addresses the views of those within a group but does not address how those outside a particular group might interpret the same knowledge. Rather, the purpose of this book is to give life to the voices of members of populations themselves.

Genetics and identity

Lastly, and perhaps most importantly, this book addresses the impact of genetic knowledge on Jewish self-identity. There has been much discussion on the potential of new genetic knowledge to significantly alter and transform social arrangements, individual identity and concepts of kinship and relatedness (Brodwin 2002, Finkler 2001, Hallowell 1999, Novas and Rose 2000, Rabinow 1996, Rapp 2000, Strathern 1992). Rabinow (1996) coined the term 'biosociality' to refer to the ways in which genetics will reshape society and identity, and individuals may come to identify themselves and their community through their genes and biology. Biosociality has been very widely referenced by social scientists 'mapping and investigating the transformations in knowledge and identity brought about by new genetic knowledge' (Gibbon and Novas 2007: 1). Rabinow's (1996) observations were based on research in France in the early 1990s, when patients, relatives and others affected by a group of diseases known as dystrophics mobilized and became actively involved in the search for treatments and a cure. They significantly affected research and successfully lobbied for funding to be directed towards their neglected disease. Biosociality will be evident in the ways in which Ashkenazi Jews advocated for Tay-Sachs screening (chapter one) and later developments related to BRCA genetic breast cancer (chapter two).

For Novas and Rose (2000: 485), advances in genetics and genetic medicine are leading to a 'mutation in personhood' with many implications for how individuals conceive of themselves and their bodies. Individuals may obtain a genetic status and as a result may feel a genetic responsibility to take certain actions in relation to their family, their personal health, their children and many other aspects of their life. Those engaged in these activities are 'biological citizens' who 'partake in an ethic of active citizenship ... in which the maximization of lifestyle, potential, health, and quality of life has become almost obligatory' (Rose 2007: 25). For Finkler (2000), current genetic developments have led to a resurgence of the biological importance of kin and family especially in relation to genetic disease, thereby leading to a return to notions of kinship based on consanguinity rather than choice. Her work follows that of Strathern (1992), for example, who has shown the ways in which Western reproductive technologies are reconfiguring reproduction and kinship processes assumed to be 'natural' or 'biological'. Importantly, genetic knowledge can reinforce older categories or notions of group belonging, particularly if such knowledge fits with pre-existing narratives (Brodwin 2002, Prainsack 2007, Rabinow 1996).

There have been criticisms that genetic research specific to Ashkenazi Jews could lead to a belief that collective identity is the result of biological as opposed to social mechanisms (Azoulay 2003, Brodwin 2002, Kahn 2005). For Brodwin (2002), emerging genetic knowledge has the potential to transform contemporary notions of individual and collective identity and lead to the idea of biologically fixed racial identities and differences. These discussions tend to assume that current genetics will have negative consequences for the collective identity of Jews by causing individuals to think of identity in terms of biology and genetics, while simultaneously assuming it is possible to delineate 'social' and 'biological' identities, something that this book will show is not an accurate reflection of how people experience their Jewish identity. By exploring women's experiences of being Jewish and at increased risk of genetic breast cancer, this book directly addresses whether knowing that the increased risk of genetic breast cancer is associated with being Jewish has an impact on how women feel about their own Ashkenazi Jewish identity. What role does biology play in what 'being Jewish' means, especially in a context where being Jewish also confers an increased risk of disease? As we will see, biological discourses are an important part of Jewish self-identity and genetic knowledge does not necessarily transform or alter identity but can in fact reiterate collective identity, particularly if it fits with pre-existing narratives and concerns. Genetic breast cancer and mutations can lead women to recall collective history, provide connections to common ancestors and origins, reiterate interrelatedness, while also having implications for the survival of future generations. The topic of Jewish identity is huge and not a monolithic whole and in this research I have focused specifically on the impact that being at increased risk of genetic disease might have on how people conceive of their own Jewish belonging.

The subject of Jewish identity, including the question of who is a Jew and what constitutes 'Jewishness', is one of the most vexed and contested issues of modern religious and ethnic group history (Glenn and Sokoloff 2010). There is a long history of debate within Judaism about the nature of Judaism and whether it is the product of religious observance or being born Jewish (Kahn 2005). Many Ashkenazi Jews view themselves as belonging to a social or religious group brought together by common practices or history, and the notion that Jewishness is not biological has retained great cultural force especially after the Holocaust (Kahn 2005). At the same time, matrilineal descent is another important aspect that defines Jewish belonging, and the necessity of being born to a Jewish mother imbues Judaism with a biological aspect, as does the existence of supposedly 'Jewish' genetic diseases. These potentially contradictory ways of defining Jewish belonging form the basis of chapter four, but examining Ashkenazi Jewish belonging and identity highlights the inseparability and co-production (Jasanoff 2004) of the biological and social.

Throughout this book, some recurring (and familiar) themes that have populated the social science literature on the new genetics continue to arise, such as biosociality (Rabinow 1996) and co-production (Jasanoff 2004). Jasanoff's (2004) concept of co-production is especially instructive. According to Jasanoff (2004), much explanatory power is gained by thinking of natural and social orders as being produced together. Rather than a theoretical framework, Jasanoff (2004) refers to co-production as an idiom – a way of interpreting and accounting for complex phenomena. Importantly, the co-productionist framework is symmetrical and does not give primacy to either nature or society; instead it investigates the continual changes to the boundaries between the social and the natural (Jasanoff 2004: 20). Rabinow's (1996: 99) concept of biosociality also calls into question what is assumed to be natural and posits that the nature/culture split will be dissolved, with nature being remade and becoming artificial just as culture becomes natural. For Rabinow (1996) biosociality is an inversion of sociobiological thinking which suggests there is a biological or natural basis to human behaviour, culture and the social order. What these concepts, and this book, share as a common thread is that they question the boundaries, or lack thereof, between the 'biological/natural' and the 'social/cultural'.[6] Anthropology has long debated these shifting boundaries, including the ways in which the new genetics is remodelling or challenging these divisions even further (Casper and Koenig 1996, Franklin 1995, Martin 1998, Strathern 1992). Genetics reveals the labyrinthine intermingling of the realms nature/culture, calling into question both categories (Goodman et al. 2003: 5). Examining Ashkenazi Jewish identity, genetic disease and medicine is a particularly illustrative example of the inseparability of natural and social orders. In the first half of the book, this will be evident in the very development of genetic medicine itself. For example, genetic disease is a result of the demographic and social history of Ashkenazi Jews. Ashkenazi Jews have been both subjects and drivers of genetic research and screening, which can address culturally salient issues such as the survival of future generations. In the second half of the book, the question of what it means to be Jewish yet again reveals the inseparability of biological and social discourses, but this time in terms of how Jewish identity and belonging are conceptualized.

In the following section I discuss genetic breast cancer and its testing and management in the UK, before turning to the research sites and methods used.

BRCA genetic breast cancer

The vast majority of breast cancer is sporadic and age is the most important risk factor, with approximately 80 per cent of breast cancers being diagnosed after the age of 50. Approximately 5–10 per cent of all breast cancers are believed to be genetic, and about half of these are a result of mutations in the BRCA1 or BRCA2 genes (National Cancer Institute 2011). The BRCA1 gene was discovered in 1994 and is located on chromosome 17 (Miki et al. 1994). Mutations in BRCA1 confer an increased lifetime risk of up to 85 per cent for breast cancer and 40 per cent for ovarian cancer (Antoniou et al. 2003). The BRCA2 gene was identified in 1995 and is located on chromosome 13 (Wooster et al. 1995). Mutations in BRCA2 confer up to 45 per cent lifetime risk for breast cancer and 11 per cent for ovarian cancer (Wooster et al. 1995).

Genetic breast cancer usually occurs in families where there is a very strong family history of many female relatives, and sometimes males, having developed breast and/or ovarian cancer, often at a young age. However, only 25 per cent of high-risk families are found to have a mutation in either BRCA1 or 2 and there are other genes believed to contribute to the cancers in these families (Antoniou et al. 2003). There has been little progress in explaining the missing heritability for the remaining 75 per cent of those with family histories in whom no BRCA mutation is found (Ziogas et al. 2011).

Shortly after the discovery of the BRCA genes, clinical genetic testing became widely available in North America, Israel and many Western European countries (Narod 2009). In the UK, women with family histories of breast cancer can be referred to one of 24 regional genetic centres, where they are seen for an assessment of their risk and possible advice regarding genetic testing. Genetic testing is available free of charge through the National Health Service (NHS) as long as individuals meet the high-risk criteria set by the National Institute for Health and Clinical Excellence (NICE) and there is a living affected relative to provide a blood sample for genetic testing. NICE published revised guidelines in 2005 for the management of familial breast cancer and Ashkenazi Jewish ancestry was added as an important risk factor for the assessment of genetic risk. Clinicians are advised to find out if a woman has Ashkenazi Jewish ancestry and include this in their decision to make a referral to a local genetic centre.

National context has affected the 'architecture' of genetic testing for breast cancer very differently, as Parthasarathy's (2007) comparison of the US and UK has shown. In the United States a private company called Myriad is the sole commercial provider of BRCA genetic testing. During the 1990s there was a furious race by several international academic and commercial teams to clone the BRCA1 and BRCA2 genes. Myriad won the race (Goldstein 2008) and subsequently filed a series of patents based on the sequence of the genes and obtained a monopoly on all BRCA genetic testing in the United States. This monopoly has kept the cost of the test relatively high (up to 3,000 US dollars). Despite early attempts by Myriad to enforce their patents in Europe, challenges and subsequent decisions by the European Patent Office (EPO) have eroded most of Myriad's patents outside the United States. In the UK testing is performed by National Health Service accredited laboratories (at a much lower cost) despite early threats by Myriad to sue the National Health Service. Myriad's lack of success in enforcing their patents outside the United States led them to attempt to enforce only their patents for the three 'Ashkenazi mutations' in Europe, and in June 2005 the EPO upheld this decision. This ruling technically meant that only Ashkenazi Jewish patients in Europe would have to pay for BRCA mutation testing through Myriad. Most European labs simply refused to abide by this ruling, which was considered 'racial discrimination', so this practice has not been implemented in the UK or Europe (Abbott 2005: 12). Israeli geneticists claimed that charging only one ethnic group for a particular test or procedure was racist and violated fundamental tenets of equality (Goldstein 2008). The attempt by Myriad to enforce only their patents for the Ashkenazi mutations points to a larger concern regarding the potentially discriminatory, unequal and unjust ways in which commercialized genetic medicine can develop in relation to different populations.

More recently Myriad has become headline news again due to a legal suit brought against it by the American Civil Liberties Union which claims that the patents stifle diagnostic testing and research and are therefore unconstitutional. The case is still ongoing and may go before the Supreme Court, particularly as it has reopened a much more fundamental debate about whether genes should be patentable at all. As women in the UK are able to access BRCA testing free of charge through the National Health Service, the Myriad story does not form a significant part of this book or of individual women's stories, but this may not be the case in other countries or contexts where issues such as access to, and the cost of, health care are more pressing.

Management options

There are two main management options for BRCA mutation carriers or women at high genetic risk: increased surveillance and prophylactic surgery. Carriers can opt for surveillance through annual mammography in an attempt to detect breast cancer at an early stage when treatment has a higher success rate. However, there is data that suggests increased exposure to radiation as a result of early mammography may itself increase the risk of breast cancer (Bankhead et al. 2001). Screening can lead to increased anxiety before, during and after the appointment while awaiting results. Breast tissue is especially dense in younger women, making mammograms more difficult to interpret and increasing the chance of false positives where a woman is recalled for a repeat mammogram or biopsy. As a result, NICE (2005) now recommends breast screening with magnetic resonance imaging (MRI) for young women who are at high risk, although this is a more costly option which may not be available in poorer developing countries (Narod 2009). Alternately, women can opt for prophylactic mastectomy. Surgically removing both breasts significantly reduces the chance of developing breast cancer (by about 90 per cent) but does not eliminate the risk entirely and comes with considerable psychosocial adverse effects (Ziogas et al. 2011). According to an evidence review by NICE (2005), prophylactic mastectomy should be very carefully considered before being offered and must take place with the help and care of a multi-disciplinary team that includes psychological support for the woman. Hormonal treatment with a drug called Tamoxifen is also available and has been shown to prevent the development of breast cancer in some women. However, screening and prophylactic surgery remain the two most common management options for women at significant genetic risk.

Management options for the increased risk of ovarian cancer present a more complicated picture as there is no proven effective screening method for early detection, although research studies are under way. There are no national guidelines or screening methods currently available to detect the disease. The symptoms are notoriously hard to detect and by the time it is diagnosed the cancer has very often spread and is at a late stage. Five year survival for ovarian cancer is very low as a result (Cancer Research UK 2008). Prophylactic oophorectomy (surgical removal of the ovaries) is recommended for mutation carriers, especially as it may also decrease the risk of breast cancer (Haber 2002). As BRCA mutations confer an increased risk of cancer at a young age (below 50), prophylactic removal of the ovaries may be a particularly difficult decision for younger women as it prevents childbearing and induces menopause.

There is no absolutely reliable method of early diagnosis or prevention for breast or ovarian cancer, and this can leave women with lifelong fears about developing cancer (Mor and Oberle 2008: 516). There is a relatively substantial body of research related to BRCA which is primarily psychosocial and has focused on the affective psychological implications of genetic testing on individuals, although not specifically Ashkenazi Jews (Cox and McKellin 1999, Hallowell et al. 1997, Lodder et al. 1999, 2001, Watson et al. 2004). Much of the evidence, including a systematic review, has shown no adverse psychological consequences such as anxiety, anger, guilt or depression as a result of testing (Broadstock et al. 2000, Lerman et al. 1996, Schwartz et al. 2002, Watson et al. 1996). There is, however, evidence to the contrary which has shown that some individuals experience increased levels of anxiety and distress post-test result (Croyle et al. 1997, Lodder et al. 2001, Lynch et al. 1997, Michie et al. 2001). There have been few follow-up studies beyond one year to document the long-term consequences of BRCA testing and the knowledge that one is a mutation carrier or at significantly increased risk of developing cancer in the future.

There is very little empirical data regarding the implications and perceptions of BRCA testing among Ashkenazi Jews (Lehman et al. 2002, Phillips et al. 2000, Rothenberg 2000). Previous studies have utilized standardized questionnaires or telephone interviews to primarily address concerns regarding discrimination. The results confirm that, despite some concerns, there appears to be a highly supportive attitude towards genetic research and testing. However, these studies are not qualitative and do not explore the impact that knowledge of genetic disease may have on Jewish identity.

Research methods and sites

This book is the result of multiple methods carried out at multiple sites, including participant observation, in-depth interviews, placements in genetic laboratories, a quantitative survey and professional experience in BRCA clinical research. Between 2002 and 2010 I worked in an academic clinical trials unit where I managed and helped develop research studies specifically related to breast and ovarian cancer genetics, including a national ovarian cancer screening study and a chemotherapy clinical trial for BRCA mutation carriers. This work brought me into contact with many BRCA carriers, high-risk women, clinicians and scientists working in the field. Of particular relevance is the fact that I was responsible for a separately funded Israeli research collaboration with the aim of maximizing the number of Ashkenazi women with BRCA mutations recruited to the chemotherapy clinical trial. Recruiting Ashkenazi Jews was essential to reaching the total number of study participants required and highlights the importance of this population from a clinical and research point of view. This work included involving BRCA carriers in the design of clinical research and I organized consultation panels, created patient videos, websites and patient information specifically for BRCA mutation carriers.

In addition to my professional role, the primary research methods were participant observation and qualitative interviews with high-risk Ashkenazi women attending two NHS clinics located in central London – a cancer genetics clinic and a family history clinic. These clinics provided a fairly accessible way of identifying women who were at increased risk and considering genetic testing. One result of choosing this site is that I did not have access to those who were refusing to come forward for genetic testing. It is possible that some women may not come forward because of discomfort about being singled out as Ashkenazi Jews, and therefore the women I encountered may have had fewer concerns about research since they had already sought out genetic services. At both clinics I observed clinical consultations between genetic counsellors or family history nurses and consenting women. Following the consultation, I would ask women if they were interested in taking part in a separate in-depth interview. A total of 14 interviews with high-risk women were carried out. Interviews took place in women's homes (n = 10), in a university office (n = 3) and on one occasion in a coffee shop. The majority of the women were British or American Jews between 25 and 75 years of age and were in professional or semi-professional occupations, graduate students, stay-at-home mothers or retired. Most were secular (n = 12) and two were ritually observant. Some women had breast cancer while others only had a family history of the disease. All the women were considered to be at increased risk and eligible for BRCA genetic testing under UK National Health Service guidelines, although not all had undergone testing. Only one woman interviewed was a known BRCA mutation carrier.

During interviews I had a rough topic guide with the issues that I wanted to cover, but I was very flexible and I let the interviews evolve naturally as 'conversations with a purpose' (Byrne 2004: 181). I found that it was more useful to allow people to tell me what they thought was important to them, rather than forcing particular questions on individuals. However, in all interviews we talked about Jewish identity, Jewish upbringing and what role Judaism played in women's lives currently, women's family histories, or personal experiences, of breast cancer and their understanding and feelings about the genetic risk being higher for Ashkenazi Jewish women. Interviews generally lasted one to two hours but sometimes extended over an entire afternoon or a whole day, and I felt that I came to know many of the women well. All interviews except one, where the interviewee declined, were digitally recorded and transcribed.

Given the diversity of the Ashkenazi Jewish women attending the clinics, it is not possible or desirable to make generalizations about the women interviewed other than that no ultra-Orthodox women were interviewed. The reason for not interviewing any ultra-Orthodox was partly practical as very few were referred to either of the clinics I attended, and one genetic counsellor told me that she believed most were seen privately and not in the NHS. However, I did not seek out any ultra-Orthodox women because they are a unique and discrete group with very strong religious affiliation who are generally removed from the secular world. This research focuses on those for whom Judaism played less of a role in their lives to see whether genetic knowledge affected how they thought about being Jewish. The ultra-Orthodox are also a minority of Jews, and while this research is not representative of any particular 'community' of Jews, it reflects the diversity of modern Jews, many of whom are secular.

Women were extremely open and generous with me, sharing private experiences and allowing me into their lives and homes. An important factor that made it possible for me to explore women's personal stories is my own role in this research as a secular, unmarried Ashkenazi Jewish woman. Although I have no family history of breast cancer, my identity provided a level of trust and comfort that allowed women to be open with me. They usually wanted to confirm that I was Jewish and our interviews very often felt like an intimate conversation between two Jewish women who were sharing experiences. This was an advantage rather than a hindrance. Kahn (2000) has discussed the implications of being a Jewish woman doing an ethnography of Jews. She points out that her critical stance is inevitably informed by her identification with the collectivity she has chosen to study, and more importantly their identification with her as 'one of them' (Kahn 2000: 5). While compelling ethnography has more to do with the degree of identification between the ethnographer and her subject, Kahn's dual status as insider and outsider offered her a unique opportunity. This is also true of my own research, as I believe that a non-Jewish woman would not have engendered the same level of comfort and safety that allowed women to share their stories and feelings with me.

In addition, I carried out participant observation and in-depth interviews with non-high-risk individuals in parts of the Jewish 'community' in North London. Although it does not represent a single unified 'community' of Jews, North London has the highest proportion of Jews in the UK (Levene 2005) and, as a secular and Canadian Jew who is not affiliated with any Jewish organizations or synagogues, the London Jewish Cultural Centre was one particular accessible location in North London where I was able to meet other Jews and attend events that were specifically designed for the Jewish communities in this part of London. I attended lectures, talks, courses and events over an 18-month period, many of which were about Jewish identity, belonging or genetics. I interviewed five individuals that I met at the London Jewish Cultural Centre, including four men. The purpose of these interviews was to discuss Jewish identity and belonging, as well as the level of awareness individuals had about genetic disease and research related to Jews. The individuals who were not at risk often had no direct experience and very little knowledge of genetic disease and, despite having heard of Tay Sachs, this made further probing about this topic rather difficult. This provides evidence that, for people without any direct experience of genetic disease, it is not a significant factor in their own identity or daily life. However, the voices of the non-high-risk individuals, including the men, are included throughout the book, particularly regarding Jewish identity (chapter four) and endogamy (chapter six).

Following a careful reading of the transcripts and field notes, data was analysed and coded using qualitative thematic analysis (Seale 2004: 313) for categories and themes that arose repeatedly. The coding scheme emerged deductively and inductively from the data itself, and this highlights the importance of exploratory research that can reveal previously unanticipated issues (Seale 2004). All names and personal identifiers have been changed.

The qualitative and ethnographic methods were supplemented by a quantitative self-completed postal survey. The survey provides data on the knowledge a non-high-risk group had regarding the BRCA mutations and contributes to overcoming the lack of information on awareness levels in the general Jewish population. The survey included questions about religious identity, familiarity with genetic disease and testing, cancer history and a series of eight BRCA knowledge questions, one of which asked if people were aware of the increased risk for Ashkenazi Jews. Over 200 questionnaires were distributed through Jewish organizations, Jewish events and university departments in London. The survey had a response rate of over 50 per cent, with 111 returned. All survey respondents were asked for permission to be contacted in future to take part in an in-depth interview. Although the survey data does not form a large part of the analysis, it provides the only data on BRCA awareness among a non-high-risk population of Ashkenazi Jews (discussed in chapter three).

Lastly, I also benefited from spending time in two human genetic laboratories, including a high throughput BRCA sequencing laboratory where I carried out basic lab work. Although this book is not an ethnographic study of laboratory practice, which has a well established history within anthropology and other social science disciplines (Fujimura 1996, Latour and Woolgar 1979, Rabinow 1996, Rapp 2000), I did benefit from the ongoing interaction with scientists and my increased understanding of what goes on in the day-to-day workings of a genetic laboratory. The laboratory placements and interaction with scientists also forced me to face my own disciplinary deficiencies and at times jargon-filled, confusing language. I have attempted throughout this book to write in language that is clear and can be understood across the disciplinary divides. I also became aware of the highly critical nature of some social science writing about genetics and scientists that did not seem to accurately reflect my own experience in the lab or working with scientists and clinicians. The implication, perhaps unintended, of some critical social science writing is that scientists are somehow deliberately distancing themselves from the social aspects of their work and this can have the effect of alienating scientists and creating acrimony. According to Franklin (1995), the fact that scientists so vehemently defend science is a sign that science is cultural and its beliefs are deeply held. While this may be true, I have come to feel defensive of scientists and careful about the claims I make. I believe this is one of the major benefits of interdisciplinary work in that it allows social scientists and scientists to interact and question and learn about each other's disciplinary standpoints.

Book outline

Genetic knowledge has an inevitable temporal aspect that links individuals to their familial and collective past, to the present and to future generations (see Finkler 2000). This temporality has become an organizing theme for the chapters. The story begins by looking back at early genetic screening programmes for Tay-Sachs and also at how genetic mutations and disease can become linked with collective Jewish history (chapter one). The book then moves to the present, where the Ashkenazi BRCA mutations, advocacy and the implications of genetic breast cancer risk for Jewish self-identity are explored (chapters two, three and four). Genetic breast cancer also leads women to recall individual family and collective histories (chapter five). Lastly, the book examines the future and in particular the consequences of genetic knowledge for future generations (chapter six). As Margaret Lock (1998) accurately notes, genetic testing for breast cancer permits us to divine our past and to make that heritage – in the form of genes – into omens for the future. Below I provide a more detailed outline of each chapter.

Chapter one describes the history and background to the involvement of Ashkenazi Jews in medical genetic research and screening programmes, in particular for Tay-Sachs disease. The chapter also discusses some of the reasons for this historical participation in and support of genetic research, including Jewish theology, history and cultural factors. Genetic disease is linked with collective Jewish history and suffering, and genetic medicine can become a mechanism to address culturally salient issues. This chapter helps to contextualize and reveal the interconnections with the current developments related to BRCA described in chapter two. Two continuities between Tay-Sachs research and screening are drawn out in chapter two. The first is the way in which the 'Ashkenazi BRCA mutations' are associated with collective Jewish history and suffering, and the second is the role of Ashkenazi Jews as advocates for BRCA genetic research and screening, which may be partially explained by the ways in which genetic mutations and disease reflect and reiterate Jewish collective identity and history. However, there may be unintended consequences to participating in research, such as becoming over-represented, leading to increasing numbers of diseases being labelled as 'Jewish' as a result.

Chapter three turns to the specific criticisms about genetic research focused on Ashkenazi Jews. Rather than relying on the 'lessons of history' to warn against the potential harms of current genetics, this chapter takes a different approach by exploring whether individuals had concerns about research or saw it as a continuation of historical discrimination. Individuals do not necessarily interpret current genetics as an extension of historical forms of anti-Semitism or eugenics. At the same time, there was evidence that women did have a heightened and inaccurate belief that all Ashkenazi women were at increased risk of breast cancer, and clinical encounters, physicians and family history questionnaires could all reinforce this sense of risk. While this may not have been a problem for women themselves, who mostly believed it was essential to promote awareness, it does raise questions about how others, especially non-Jews, might interpret the same information.

Chapter four specifically examines the impact that knowledge of genetic breast cancer risk has on Jewish identity. The chapter begins with a discussion of the ways in which identity and kinship are conceptualized within Judaism, and then uses interview material to show how individuals conceptualized their own Jewish identity and belonging. Was it seen as a cultural or biological identity? Does being at increased risk of genetic disease affect how people think about their own Jewishness? Is there compatibility between new genetic knowledge and the pre-existing ways in which Jewish identity is conceived? This chapter challenges the existing literature on the impact of genetic knowledge on identity by providing evidence of the way in which genetic disease can reiterate individual and collective identity, while demonstrating the co-production (Jasanoff 2004) and inseparability of biological and social notions of Jewish belonging.

Chapter five explores how the transmission of genetic breast cancer and mutations can convey individual memory and reaffirm collective history. In the context of genetic breast cancer, family history tracing necessitates recalling those in previous generations, and for some women with strong family histories there was evidence of a tendency to 'forget' and at times silence these histories so that genetic disease not only conveyed, but also suppressed, memory. This lack of remembering appeared to be a strategy to deal with the significant anxieties and worries that women had about their risk. This chapter highlights the need for caution as Ashkenazi women may potentially face unnecessary and increased levels of anxiety, especially if they are more frequently identified as 'high risk' and referred to genetic clinical services. Chapter six turns to the implications of BRCA mutations for future generations, and the genetic responsibility individuals felt to protect their daughters and future generations of Jews from inheriting BRCA mutations and developing genetic breast cancer. The chapter focuses on the temporal nature of women's accounts that located responsibility (and at times blame) for genetic disease in the collective reproductive history of Ashkenazi Jews, and currently among specific groups of Ashkenazi Jews, namely the ultra-Orthodox. This knowledge can have potential future reproductive consequences, and a contradiction may arise between a pre-existing sense of responsibility to produce future generations of Jews and a responsibility to produce future breast-cancer-free children.

The conclusion draws together the evidence from the data presented in the previous chapters to discuss the overall findings of this research and how they support, extend and contradict some of the major concerns regarding genetic research, identity and populations. Areas for future research are also discussed.

1 Setting the scene

Ashkenazi Jews and genetic disease

> Giving life to new individual bodies, finding cures for the sick, improving the human race, grants the survival of the collective body.
>
> (Prainsack and Firestine 2006: 41)

Ashkenazi Jews are the most researched population and are over-represented in human genetic literature, especially in mutation related contexts (Birenbaum Carmeli 2004). As the population geneticist David Goldstein (2008) notes, a quick search of the literature on the biomedical search engine pubmed retrieves more than 1,300 papers about Ashkenazi Jews and genetic disease. Ashkenazi Jews are believed to have a unique and supportive relationship with medical genetics. How can this be explained? Are Jews more ill than other people? Are scientists and doctors more interested in Jews? Are Jews particularly supportive of genetics? Many questions are raised by their proliferation within research, and in order to unpack this relationship it is necessary to look back and examine the historical involvement of Ashkenazi Jews with medical genetics. This chapter focuses on Tay-Sachs disease, which can be thought of as the archetypal and original 'Ashkenazi Jewish genetic disease'. Tay-Sachs screening programmes were the first large-scale voluntary screening effort for reproductive-aged individuals in any population and for any genetic disease (Kaback 2000). Although Tay-Sachs is very different from genetic breast cancer, understanding how Tay-Sachs was discovered, its connection to Jewish history and the role of Jews in advocating for research and screening provides a framework for examining the more recent developments related to BRCA genetics and allows us to see the continuities and interconnections between them.

The chapter begins with an explanation of why Ashkenazi Jews are considered a 'population' from a genetic standpoint and why they figure so prominently in research. In particular, I focus on the ways in which genetic diseases specific to Ashkenazi Jews can become linked with Jewish history and issues that are culturally salient for Jews, and the role of Jewish advocacy in the development of Tay-Sachs research and screening programmes. The last part of the chapter discusses other contributing factors, such as Jewish theology and the political and cultural context, that help to explain why Ashkenazi

Jews may be particularly supportive and participatory in genetic research and screening programmes. This chapter highlights the 'social' nature of genetic medicine and I will make particular use of Jasanoff's (2004) concept of co-production, that is, thinking of natural and social orders as being produced together. The co-production of the biological and social will be evident in terms of the explanations for the origins of genetic disease among Ashkenazi Jews, how they have come to be so represented in research and their participation in and advocacy for research and testing.

What is a population?

From the perspective of genetics, populations are groups who are genetically differentiated from one another because of geographical and/or cultural isolation (Burchard et al. 2003). Historically, genetic differentiation occurred largely because of geographic barriers, such as mountains, deserts or large bodies of water, which restricted mating and reproduction between people. This means that genetic differentiation often occurs between continentally separated groups, although cultural practices such as endogamy, religion and language have given rise to even further genetic subdivisions within continents (Burchard et al. 2003). This is known as 'assortative mating' and refers to the non-random choice of partners based on characteristics such as geographical proximity, skin colour, height or religion (Bamshad et al. 2004). Over time, these reproductive patterns result in greater genetic homogeneity than for those populations who intermarry and mate with one another (Bittles 2005). While populations are fluid and not fixed biologically, they may differ from one another genetically. Populations are never entirely reproductively closed and there will always be mating between and across groups. The mixing of two or more populations who are genetically differentiated from one another is known as 'admixture' (Bamshad et al. 2004). Genetic differentiation is therefore caused by physical conditions such as geography as well as factors such as religion, cultural practices and language. Isolation of populations can also be a result of discrimination, stigmatization and overt political efforts which force certain groups into isolation. In the case of Ashkenazi Jews this is particularly relevant, as they have a history of discrimination and the existence of genetic disease can become linked with their history of oppression and suffering.

Populations are important for medical genetics because of their presumed genetic homogeneity, which makes them easier to study in a laboratory as there may be fewer variables which need to be controlled for and because it is easier to detect genetic variation that is statistically more likely to be related to the trait of interest (M'Charek 2005, Montoya 2007). Isolated populations help to understand disease in genetically diverse and complex populations because they act as 'control populations' against which the diverse populations can be compared. The availability of detailed multi-generational genealogies and environmental similarities also contribute to their utility (Arcos 2002). Thus, they fit neatly into a scientific laboratory method wherein as many uncontrollable variables as possible are removed (M'Charek 2005). As Marks (2008) explains, the current conception of population involves looking at the most divergent qualities of the most geographically separated groups (basically those at the extremes) in order to maximize detectable difference. Importantly, isolated populations may also have an increased incidence of certain inherited diseases, which is believed to be the result of the processes of genetic drift and the founder effect.

Genetic drift

Whereas natural selection presumes that beneficial alleles will increase in frequency over time, genetic drift is the random fluctuation in the frequency of a specific gene or allele in a population regardless of whether it is beneficial or not (Stone et al. 2007).[1] According to genetic drift, there is always a possibility that a deleterious genetic mutation will survive randomly. Genetic drift is inversely related to population size so that in a small population genetic drift will have a stronger effect (Bamshad et al. 2004). If, for example, one member of a founding population carries a deleterious mutation but the founding population contains 1,000 members, then only 0.1 per cent of the total population carries the mutation and the effect is not particularly large. If, on the other hand, the founding population has only 10 members, then 10 per cent of the population is now affected with the mutation and so the 'genetic drift' has a much larger influence.

The founder effect

The founder effect is a process of genetic drift that results from a founder event. A founder event occurs when a population has a small number of founding ancestors who are separated from the larger parent population and go on to found a new population (Stone et al. 2007). Alternatively, a founder event can be the result of an extreme reduction of a population, by over 50 per cent, due to famine, war, epidemic or some other event that causes a significant number of a population's members to die. This is known as population bottleneck because the population suddenly contracts. In both of these situations, the new founding population carries only a fraction of the original population's genetic variation and is not representative of the entire diverse population from which it was derived but only a small portion of it (Goldstein 2008, Stone et al. 2007). As a result this new population can be quite distinct from the original population. The founder effect occurs when at least one of the members of the new founding population carries a genetic mutation which is then passed on to future generations. The mutation may substantially increase in frequency if the population remains reproductively closed, for example due to cultural practices such as endogamy. Members of founding populations tend to live in close geographic proximity and so are more likely to mate with one another, which will increase the frequency of the mutation as the population increases in size (Bamshad et al. 2004).

Selective advantage

In contrast to genetic drift, which is random, there may be a beneficial effect to carrying a single copy of a mutated allele, which explains its high frequency in a given population. For example, carrying a single copy of the sickle cell allele provides resistance to malaria. Some argue that the fact that Tay-Sachs has remained within the Ashkenazi population at such a high frequency is evidence that it must have a selective advantage, and it has been proposed that carrying a copy of the Tay-Sachs allele could provide immunity from tuberculosis, something that would have been advantageous in the ghettos of Eastern Europe (Cochran et al. 2005, Goodman 1979). Most of the diseases that occur at increased incidence among Ashkenazi Jews are recessive and recessive diseases could provide a selective advantage because carrying a single copy of the gene does not cause disease. The fact that many of the diseases that occur among Ashkenazi Jews relate to the central nervous system has been taken as further evidence that these mutations cannot just be the result of genetic drift and the founder effect but must provide a selective advantage. The issue has been debated for over 40 years and remains unresolved. However, Risch et al. (2003: 812) claim that there is strong and compelling evidence to support genetic drift over selection as the primary determinant of disease mutations in the Ashkenazi population.

Founder effect, genetic drift and Ashkenazi Jewish history

Ashkenazi Jews are those Jews who originate from Eastern and Central Europe. Although the word Ashkenazi actually means German, it has come to mean Eastern Europe because most Jews were concentrated there between the tenth and nineteenth centuries. Although they are now dispersed throughout the world, approximately 80 per cent of the world's Jewish population is of Ashkenazi origin (Markel 1997). All Jews originated in the Middle East but, following the destruction of the second temple in around 70 CE, many fled and were dispersed out of the Middle East (Goldstein 2008). Many of these Jews settled in Europe and while it is not entirely clear when they first arrived, there are records of Jews in France and Germany dating from the fourth century CE. Jews in Western Europe faced increasing persecution and were legally expelled from some countries, including England in 1290 and France in 1394 (Markel 1997). Beginning in the eleventh century, many began to flee to Eastern Europe, especially Poland, Lithuania and Russia, where they initially faced less persecution. This early Jewish migration to Eastern Europe consisted of many small groups, often just a few families who settled in isolated areas. These families were isolated genetically from their non-Jewish neighbours as well as other small Jewish settlements (Goodman 1979).

By the end of the sixteenth century, Poland had the largest Jewish population in Europe and was the major centre of the Jewish world (Markel 1997). Even as the population grew, Jews in Eastern Europe continued to live in isolation from the surrounding non-Jewish culture. They spoke a different language – Yiddish – and lived in small towns or villages called shtetls. Anti-Semitism was increasing in Eastern Europe throughout the sixteenth and seventeenth centuries, so Jews began to move back to Western Europe where many of the prior legal bans restricting them had been removed. The last ban on Jews was revoked in England in 1656. By the early nineteenth century, a series of increasingly anti-Jewish laws exiled most Eastern European Jews to particular districts in western Russia and eastern Poland which became known as the Pale of Settlement. These laws restricted Jews from travelling outside the Pale and limited their business dealings and religious rituals, barred them from universities and enforced conscription into the Russian army. By 1897, 94 per cent of the entire Russian Jewish population lived in the Pale, which severely isolated them from the surrounding culture and people. This social separation fitted well with pre-existing Jewish traditions that called for complete separation from the secular non-Jewish world (Markel 1997). Initially, the relative absence of war and improved health conditions within the Pale allowed the population to significantly grow for three generations (Goodman 1979).

Ashkenazi Jews are ideal research subjects because their history exemplifies both the founder effect and genetic drift (Kahn 2005). They are descended from a small number of founding ancestors derived from a larger population who were restricted to one particular geographical area and then practised endogamy. Ashkenazi Jewish history also conforms to the theory of genetic drift or bottleneck because the population of Eastern European Jews was often greatly reduced as a result of famine, war or epidemic, and, as will be shown in the following chapter, the Ashkenazi BRCA mutations have been correlated with specific historical events. Jewish history is fairly well documented over the past 4,000 years in terms of migration, location and population events, providing a particularly attractive study population. Without such historical knowledge, it would be much more difficult to make conclusive genetic statements. When individuals are stripped of all prior information about ancestry, geographical origins or ethnic group, and are then assigned to groups a posteriori, racial categories or geographical origins based on genetic data become much less reliable (Bamshad et al. 2004). Without external information such as texts, oral history or archaeology, it is difficult, if not impossible, to tell a coherent story about a population based on genetic information alone (Goldstein 2008). Ashkenazi Jewish history, cultural practices and isolation in response to discrimination have given Ashkenazi Jews an increased risk of certain genetic diseases. It is this that makes them important, and particularly interesting, for population genetics and disease research. Genetic differentiation and mutations are a reflection of the particular geographic, migrational, reproductive and social histories of populations.[2] Genetic risks are therefore the result of the 'biosocial histories' of populations, which includes historical and life circumstances (Marks 2008).

Tay-Sachs: the archetypal 'Ashkenazi Jewish genetic disease'

The best-known genetic disease that occurs at increased incidence among Ashkenazi Jews is Tay-Sachs, although other diseases are prevalent. Tay-Sachs is an incurable degenerative neurological disorder of the central nervous system. Babies with Tay-Sachs are born healthy but at around six months the disease leads to a series of deteriorations including blindness, seizures, profound retardation and paralysis. Death usually occurs before the age of five and no treatment exists. Tay-Sachs was first described in 1881 by an English ophthalmologist, Dr Warren Tay, and later more fully by Dr Bernard Sachs, a neurologist in New York, in 1887 and more definitely in 1896 (Cowan 2008, Edelson 1997, Wailoo and Pemberton 2006). During the 1880s there was massive emigration to the United States by Ashkenazi Jews who were escaping the increasingly harsh living conditions and persecution they faced in the Pale of Settlement in Eastern Europe. Between 1880 and 1924 more than 2.1 million Jews immigrated to the United States, representing 33 per cent of all the Jews living in Eastern Europe at the time (Markel 1997). Early Jewish immigrants to America continued the 'shtetl' style of living in small and close knit neighbourhoods that they had established in Eastern Europe and the Pale of Settlement. They lived separated not only from non-Jews but also from one another based on geographic origins and economic status. A Russian Jew would not, for example, marry a Sephardic Jew in the early twentieth century because of their historical and/or social differences (Markel 1997). In this regard, different Jewish groups continued to remain fairly homogeneous. In the last 50 or 60 years these differentiations have disintegrated so that not only do most Jews not distinguish between other groups of Jews, but they very often assimilate and marry non-Jews. This has consequences for genetic screening programmes and will be returned to later in the chapter.

For the next 80 years or so Tay-Sachs was recognized as a rare but recurring disease primarily but not exclusively in descendants of Eastern European Jews. As the American Ashkenazi community grew, so did the incidence of Tay-Sachs. By the mid-1950s an entire ward in the hospital for chronic diseases in Brooklyn was devoted to the care of children with Tay-Sachs or similar diseases (Edelson 1997). A group of Jewish parents of children with Tay-Sachs formed the National Tay-Sachs and Allied Diseases Association in 1957 and a research institute was set up. By the mid-1960s Tay-Sachs and other related diseases were recognized as having similar biological mechanisms, and a great deal of research was carried out in relation to these 'storage diseases'. They are known as storage diseases because they lead to an abnormal storage of sphingolipids (lipids commonly found in neural tissue). In 1971 an enzyme test was developed that could identify carriers of Tay-Sachs as well as diagnose foetuses in utero, making screening of the Jewish population possible (Goodman and Goodman 1982). Since there is no cure for Tay-Sachs, efforts focused on mass screening and genetic counselling.

The first Tay-Sachs screening programme began in the Baltimore/Washington area of the United States almost as soon as testing became feasible (Goodman and Goodman 1982). Members of the American Jewish population were integral to setting up and promoting both the initial research into Tay-Sachs as well as subsequent screening programmes. Many of the initial Tay-Sachs researchers and doctors were Jewish, and according to Birenbaum Carmeli (2004) potential ethical concerns regarding genetic research into Jews may be alleviated because the researchers are Jewish. Research was also facilitated by the fact that many Jews lived in proximity to large urban medical and research centres. Funds were raised by and within the Jewish community, while rabbis and members of the community took on the role of educating Jews about Tay-Sachs and organizing screening drives. Mass mailings and television and radio advertising were used to promote the voluntary screening programme, and in the first year after Tay-Sachs screening was introduced in the United States 7,000 adults were screened, representing 10 per cent of the eligible population (Duster 1990). Raz (2010: 51) refers to the high degree of collaboration between clinical researchers and community leaders, and the role of patients in driving forward medical research and clinical agendas as 'grassroots genetics advocacy'.

Screening programmes

Tay-Sachs screening programmes now exist throughout the world, including the USA, UK, Canada, Israel, South Africa, Australia, New Zealand and the Netherlands. In the United States there are two large medical centres devoted solely to the treatment and screening of 'Jewish genetic diseases' (the Chicago Center for Jewish Genetic Disorders and the Mount Sinai Jewish Genetics Disease Center). The American Jewish Genetic Diseases Consortium represents 10 individual organizations devoted to specific Jewish genetic diseases.[3] The consortium aims to increase awareness and education about Jewish genetic diseases and encourages genetic screening for all Jews through a variety of programmes including medical grand rounds, a Rabbi education programme and Jewish community education.

Other recessive 'Ashkenazi Jewish genetic diseases' have been gradually added to these pre-existing screening programmes (Kronn et al. 1998, Levene 2005). There is no official list of 'Ashkenazi Jewish diseases' because countries differ in terms of the diseases for which screening tests are offered, but diseases that have been included in screening programmes are Tay-Sachs, Gaucher disease, Niemann-Pick type A, familial dysautonomia, cystic fibrosis, Canavan, Bloom syndrome, glycogen storage disease type 1A, mucolipidosis type IV, Fanconi anaemia group C, non-classical congenital adrenal hyperplasia, connexin 26, Usher syndrome type 1 and factor XI deficiency (Levene 2005). Not all of these diseases necessarily occur at increased incidence among Ashkenazi

Jews. Cystic fibrosis, for example, is present in the general population, but the existence of a small number of specific founder mutations among the Ashkenazi Jewish population make screening technically simpler. As a result, some countries include cystic fibrosis in their 'Ashkenazi Jewish disease' screening programmes despite the fact that Ashkenazi Jews do not have an increased risk. Most of the diseases included in screening programmes are lethal, have early childhood onset and are recessive. Recessive disorders are only manifested when two carriers have children because carrying a single copy of the allele will not cause disease. The identification of carrier status is thus a useful way of preventing disease and the basis of most screening programmes. If a couple undergoes carrier screening and neither is found to carry the recessive allele, then no action needs to be taken. If one individual is found to be a carrier, then there is no risk for the couple's children of developing the disease, but the child could inherit the recessive allele and require testing when they decide to have children in the future. If both individuals are found to be carriers, then their prospective child has a one in four chance of inheriting both copies and developing the disease. The main option for couples in this case is pre-natal screening (via amniocentesis or chorionic villus sampling) with abortion of an affected foetus, although in vitro fertilization (IVF) followed by pre-implantation genetic diagnosis (PGD), the use of donor gametes, adoption or deciding not to have children are other possible options.

In the UK, Tay-Sachs screening was approved and funded as a national screening programme within the National Health Service (NHS) in 1999, although screening had been occurring since the 1970s. UK Tay-Sachs screening was also the result of 'grassroots genetic advocacy' (Raz 2010) and was set up by Jewish parents of children who had died of Tay-Sachs and other members of the UK Jewish community. The Tay-Sachs Association was started by a taxi driver from east London whose child had died of the disease. He was angry about why he had not known about the risk and wanted to take action to raise awareness. He was helped by Emma, a warm and affec-tionate British woman in her sixties whom I interviewed. Emma had been a volunteer with the League of Jewish Women (a national voluntary welfare organization which offers help to the Jewish and wider community) for many years, and she had played a central role in the original Tay-Sachs education and screening campaigns in the UK. She also had been successfully treated for breast cancer, although she had not undergone genetic testing.

In the 1970s, while raising three children, Emma had a part-time job in a hospital. She became interested in genetics when one of her sons was born with a limb abnormality that resulted in him missing some of the fingers on his left hand, and she enrolled in a night course on genetics. The League of Jewish Women put her in contact with the taxi driver because of her interest in genetics. The two of them began to organize meetings to promote awareness of screening and distribute information to British Jews. Families from around the UK who had experience of Tay-Sachs would come to London and speak about their experiences, often in Emma's living room. Emma began to give talks in local schools and synagogues, which eventually led to the formation of the Tay-Sachs Association. Emma recalled a family from Manchester with three healthy children whose fourth was born with Tay-Sachs. This family came to London to speak about their experience; although tragic, Emma said this was also a 'blessing' because the couple particularly wanted to convey the message that even if you had numerous healthy children, there was always a possibility for two carriers that their child could be born with Tay-Sachs.

Ten years earlier, the Tay-Sachs Foundation had been started by a British Jewish man who had also lost a child to Tay-Sachs. According to Emma, this man was very wealthy and spoke to a different audience of Jews who were economically more well off. The two groups worked separately but collabora-tively and helped each other raise awareness among various parts of Jewish communities in the UK. In the 1980s both organizations wanted to promote Tay-Sachs screening via advertisements in the largest Jewish newspaper in the UK, the *Jewish Chronicle*. The Chief Rabbi at the time refused as he was concerned screening would lead to abortion, so it was only after the current Chief Rabbi, Lord Rabbi Jonathan Sacks, was appointed in 1991, that they were able to advertise more publicly in Jewish newspapers. Approximately ten years ago, all Tay-Sachs screening was taken over by the UK Jewish charity Jewish Care. Jewish Care continues to raise awareness through speaker visits to social groups, Jewish organizations, schools, clubs and hospitals, and Emma still works with this charity, giving lectures in schools and venues across London. Emma believed that much of the awareness-raising work had been successful as most Jews had now heard of Tay-Sachs, although they might not know that screening was available, and so she saw her role now as focusing primarily on the promotion of screening. According to the survey carried out as part of this research, 14 per cent of respondents had undergone genetic carrier testing for Tay-Sachs, although none of the individuals tested reported being carriers. Of the 19 in-depth qualitative interviews carried out, 18 individuals were aware of Tay-Sachs but only two had undergone testing. Almost every person I encountered throughout this research was familiar with Tay-Sachs, and it was usually the first disease individuals would mention when I asked them about genetic disease, which confirms generally high awareness levels.

Since 1970, 1.4 million individuals worldwide have undergone voluntary screening to determine if they are carriers of Tay-Sachs mutations. More than 1,400 couples have been identified as being at risk of having affected offspring (i.e. they are both carriers), and over 3,200 pregnancies have been monitored through amniocentesis or chorionic villus sampling. Of these pregnancies, 628 foetuses with Tay-Sachs have been diagnosed, and all but 19 aborted. More than 2,550 unaffected children have been born to these same families (Kaback 2000). Since the introduction of screening, the incidence of Tay-Sachs in the US and Canada has been reduced by over 90 per cent (Kaback 2000). In the UK approximately 15,000 samples have been tested for Tay-Sachs over the past 30 years, with approximately 700 tests being performed annually (Levene

2005). As a result, Tay-Sachs screening is generally hailed as a success story and has led many to consider it the prototype for other genetic screening programmes (Kaback 2000, Kronn et al. 1998, Levene 2005).

Genetic medicine can easily become entangled with community survival, and Tay-Sachs screening programmes highlight the overarching role of Jewish identity politics and the struggle for Jewish preservation in shaping genetic medicine (Wailoo and Pemberton 2006). According to Wailoo and Pemberton (2006), the early Tay-Sachs management efforts must be understood against the backdrop of Ashkenazi Jewish history, Jewish suffering and Jewish survival. Many Jewish Americans of the 1960s and 1970s were second or third generation immigrants to America who no longer lived in close knit ethnic neighbourhoods or belonged to political organizations or institutions. Jews were becoming more and more assimilated and dispersed so that symbols like the bar mitzvah became important symbols of ethnic identity.[4] As American Jews negotiated tensions between increasing assimilation and the notions of religious and cultural distinction, the idea of having distinctive diseases and 'forms of suffering' provided a powerful common reference point and a 'new form of symbolic ethnicity' (Wailoo and Pemberton 2006: 23). It is in such a context that Tay-Sachs acquired cultural significance as a Jewish disease. Scientific research into why Tay-Sachs occurs at increased incidence connects the Jewish historical past, migration patterns, the history of endogamy and insular communities in Eastern Europe with the incidence of disease, just as we will see BRCA research does in the following chapter. Even the beneficial effect theory, that being a carrier provides protection from tuberculosis, has its 'origins in the repressive social conditions of ghettos of Eastern Europe' and became symbolic of the history of Jewish oppression (Wailoo and Pemberton 2006: 25).

Over the last 50 or 60 years there has been an increasing amount of marriage between Jews and non-Jews and this has led to changes in the genetic admixture of Jewish populations, making their current homogeneity less reliable (Markel 1997). These changes have implications for genetic testing and screening programmes, especially when they are based on particular notions of population homogeneity. In September 2009 the US National Tay-Sachs and Allied Diseases Association advised that Tay-Sachs screening should return to traditional enzyme-based testing instead of the more recent use of DNA testing for specific Ashkenazi mutations, because 'the genetic mix in our society is not as segregated as it once was, so the simple DNA test may not be effective anymore' (Friedman 2010). Rising rates of intermarriage are making the Jewish population more heterogeneous, and DNA testing may miss other mutations that are prevalent in non-Jews. The change in the genetic make-up among Ashkenazi Jews is another reminder of how genetic disease incidence is a reflection of the 'biosocial' histories of this population (Marks 2008). Marks (2008: 29) suggests that human populations are best understood as 'variably sized bio-cultural units' which have their own genetic idiosyncrasies, and are historically transitory, genetically porous and culturally bounded. For Ashkenazi Jews, many studies rely on small sample numbers and the assumption that Ashkenazi Jews constitute a discrete genetically homogeneous group, with results being generalized to the entire population (Azoulay 2003, Birenbaum Carmeli 2004, Kahn 2005, Wailoo and Pemberton 2006). This ignores Ashkenazi Jews' biogenetic diversity, whether as a result of intermarriage, the markedly changing concepts of race over the last 150 years, or the social transmutability of how individuals define their origins or roots (Markel 1997: 55).

Tay-Sachs screening has not been uniformly interpreted as problem free or without its own ethical dilemmas. Goodman and Goodman (1982: 22) claim that Tay-Sachs educational campaigns for mass screening in the 1970s relied on the 'over-selling of genetic anxiety'. The campaigns attempted to motivate individuals to undergo testing through the arousal of anxiety and specifically anxiety about the Jewish history of inbreeding. Rather than discuss the founder effect, genetic drift or the possible beneficial effect of the mutations, campaigns claimed that the mutations were the result of the history of inbreeding or close marriages among Jews and so reinforced cultural stereotypes that Jews are unhealthy and inbred. According to Goodman and Goodman (1982), campaigns were manipulative and created fear in order to induce action by stressing the incurability and genetic nature of the disease. The educational materials were printed against a backdrop of the Israeli flag or the Star of David and appealed 'specifically to the values, interests, and concerns of the Jewish population toward whom [they are] ... directed' (Goodman and Goodman 1982: 22). The participation of rabbis and community leaders in the screening programmes created a conflict of interest, especially as they appeared to be endorsing the programmes while at the same they were the very people to whom Jews may turn for advice if they were uncertain about testing or abortion.

Dor Yeshorim

A unique genetic screening programme called Dor Yeshorim (Hebrew for the righteous generation) is aimed at reducing the incidence of Tay-Sachs among ultra-Orthodox Jews. Traditional ultra-Orthodox Jews (or Hasidic Jews) still undergo arranged marriages often through matchmakers, have a high birth rate (7–7.5 births/woman on average) and do not endorse abortion. I am distinguishing (albeit somewhat artificially) between the ultra-Orthodox who do not engage with the secular world and those often called Modern Orthodox who are ritually observant Jews but are not isolated from the secular world. The ultra-Orthodox do not form a single unified community and consist of many different sects and spiritual movements (Dein 2002, Raz 2010).

Dor Yeshorim began in New York in 1983 and was set up by Rabbi Joseph Ekstein, an ultra-Orthodox Rabbi who lost four of his children to Tay-Sachs. Dor Yeshorim operates by testing young members of the ultra-Orthodox community for Tay-Sachs (and now a variety of additional recessive genetic diseases) and storing the results on a centralized database. Each individual is given a number to identify themselves but is not told their results. By maintaining anonymity through non-disclosure of individual carrier status, any stigma associated with being a carrier is meant to be avoided (Prainsack and Siegal 2006). This is especially important as having a family history of genetic disease can become a serious obstacle to obtaining a marriage partner in ultra-Orthodox Jewish communities. According to the founder Rabbi Ekstein, since the primary purpose of marriage among the ultra-Orthodox is to begin a new and hopefully large family, information about the health of each partner and any potential children is of great concern, and the goal of the programme is to provide preventative measures without placing individuals at risk of social stigmatization and discrimination in the community (Ekstein and Katzenstein 2001). Traditional ultra-Orthodox Jewish matchmaking is a form of genetic selection in that the families of potential marriage partners carefully screen each other's background, including the family's history of disease, before deciding if a marriage is suitable.[5] When a potential marriage pairing is being considered, the numbers of the prospective marriage candidates are checked with the Dor Yeshorim database (by the matchmaker or the family). If both candidates are carriers, they are simply told they are not a suitable match, thus avoiding disclosure of carrier status. Dor Yeshorim requires individuals to declare they are not already engaged before the compatibility check in order to try to avoid the significant emotional costs to a couple who might find out they are not compatible, as well as any potential liability for Dor Yeshorim (Prainsack and Siegal 2006).

To date, over 120,000 individuals have been tested by Dor Yeshorim, with over 60,000 requests for 'compatibility assessments'. Over 135 potential matches have been found to be incompatible for Tay-Sachs disease, and according to Dor Yeshorim the vast majority of these incompatible couples did not pursue marriage (Ekstein and Katzenstein 2001). Virtually no children with Tay-Sachs have been born to any family who has used the database. Before the existence of Dor Yeshorim, the hospital for chronic diseases in Brooklyn had an average of 16 children with Tay-Sachs and a waiting list of children to be admitted, whereas by 1996 there were no such children in this ward. Dor Yeshorim was designed specifically to meet the 'special needs' of the Orthodox Jewish community, and the programme reflects Rabbi Ekstein's effort to translate his personal tragedy 'into a mission to spare others in his community from experiencing what he realized was *preventable*' (Ekstein and Katzenstein 2001: 301). Dor Yeshorim is an example of the way the development of a genetic screening programme can be a direct reflection of the specific religious and cultural needs of a particular group (Wailoo and Pemberton 2006).

In contrast, Raz's (2010) study of Dor Yeshorim in Israel found that it actually reinforced the stigmatization of carriers, particularly because of its insistence that individual carrier status is not disclosed, which inadvertently reinforces the message that being a carrier is something not worth knowing and ultimately 'bad'. Raz (2010) also found that while the majority of the ultra-Orthodox used Dor Yeshorim, many misunderstood the genetic basis of carrier matching (and why a match might be deemed incompatible); as a result they had a great deal of fear and held negative stigmatizing views of families with genetic disease. Dor Yeshorim has the unintended consequence of violating an individual's right to obtain information about him or herself, and by advising carrier couples not to marry it compromises widely recognized genetic counselling goals of non-directiveness and autonomy (Raz 2010).

Jewish theology and cultural context

The previous section has described the historical relationship of Ashkenazi Jews with genetic medicine, their advocacy for Tay-Sachs research and screening, and specifically how genetic diseases such as Tay-Sachs can become intertwined with Ashkenazi Jewish history. However, not all populations have had a similar trajectory in relation to genetic medicine. Ashkenazi Jews are often presented in contrast to other populations who have been less supportive or have even rejected genetic research related to them. One popular comparison is with African Americans and their rejection and distrust of much genetic research, which can broadly be traced to two particular historical events (Duster 1990, Wailoo and Pemberton 2006). The first was the Tuskegee experiments which took place in the United States between 1932 and the 1970s, and the second the sickle cell screening programmes introduced in the United States in the 1970s.[6] Mandatory sickle cell screening for all African Americans, including children, was introduced in some American states in the 1970s despite the fact that it is not fatal and has variable severity for those affected. Following mandatory testing, some carriers were unable to obtain insurance or jobs as a result of being carriers. Sickle cell screening was withdrawn as a mandatory programme because of the negative consequences and the overall distrust and lack of support by African Americans, which is a significantly different outcome from that achieved by the introduction of voluntary Tay-Sachs screening programmes during the same period. Another important difference concerns the diseases themselves. Tay-Sachs is an incurable, lethal disease that leads to a very dramatic and painful decline of babies prior to their inevitable death at a very young age. Screening is the only feasible option, especially as there has rarely been hope of a cure. Screening programmes for sickle cell were interpreted by African Americans as government attempts to limit the population, whereas Tay-Sachs screening was seen as a pronatalist act of self-preservation that could reduce the incidence of or even eliminate a severely disabling disease (Cowan 2008, Wailoo and Pemberton 2006).

How can the supportive and participatory attitude of Ashkenazi Jews in relation to genetic medicine and screening be explained? One explanation is that Jewish culture places particular value on science and medicine and that specific moral obligations create support for advancing scientific knowledge and technologies that potentially improve upon life (Prainsack and Firestine 2006, Rapp 2000, Stolberg 1998). Jewish attitudes towards health, medicine and genetics do not form a monolithic whole but comprise an assembly of various views (Prainsack and Firestine 2006), and it is not possible to make generalizations about 'Jewish' attitudes towards health and medicine, especially as there is an enormous spectrum and diversity of Jews, including those who are entirely secular. The purpose of this section is therefore not to make claims about Judaism as a whole, just as this book is not trying to make claims about 'Jews' as if they are a unified and homogeneous group. However, it is useful and important to examine the culturally specific and unique aspects, such as Jewish theology, history and political concerns, that contribute to and influence attitudes towards health, medicine and genetics.

According to Jewish theology, the body belongs to God and there is a duty to keep the body in good health and to avoid danger and injury. The duty to heal is commanded by God and medicine is viewed as an important aid in this respect. The presence of a physician is biblically required in communities of Jews, and patients are mandated to seek healing from the medical profession (Dorff 1997, Oller 1984, Rosner 2001). The duty to save one's own life and ensure good health is one of the most important commandments in Judaism, and many ancient rabbis were also part-time doctors. Unlike Christianity, Judaism has taken the stance that it is one's duty to intervene medically in 'nature' as an agent or partner of God, and violations of every Jewish law are permitted when a question of health becomes an issue (Oller 1984). The dichotomy between nature/divine creation and culture/human beings that is common in the Christian European world is not found in Jewish theology (Prainsack and Firestine 2006). Most rabbis consider scientific knowledge that will help to cure human diseases to be divinely sanctioned, if not mandated, and Jewish tradition would actually encourage Jews to find out as much about genetic diseases as they can and to participate in research in the hope of finding a cure (Dorff 1997, Rosner 2001). The ancient Talmud prohibits a man from marrying into a family where epilepsy or leprosy has appeared in case the disease is transmitted to future generations, perhaps the 'oldest recorded item of genetic counseling' (Dorff 1996: 83). The sex-linked disease haemophilia is described in the Talmud and it was forbidden to circumcise a baby if two of the baby's brothers bled to death from the procedure. Similarly, if two sisters had lost sons following circumcision, a third sister was not permitted to circumcise her baby boy, which suggests that it was recognized that females can transmit the disease but do not suffer from it (Rosner 2001).

There is a great emphasis on the duty to procreate and in most cases abortion is forbidden; however, Judaism does not view abortion as murder and it is permissible in certain circumstances (Dorff 1996). An unborn foetus is not granted the same status as a person after birth as it is regarded as part of the mother's body and not a separate being until it has emerged from the womb.[7] As a result, if the foetus threatens the mother's health or life, it must be aborted. Pregnancy is also divided into two distinct phases. Depending on the particular interpretation, within the first 40 days or the first trimester the foetus is considered simply water or 'mere fluid' (Dorff 1996, Rosner 2001).

The purpose of this demarcation is that in certain contexts abortion may be permissible. While abortion is not considered murder, it still constitutes a serious moral offence and is not encouraged as a result (Rosner 2001).

There is no justification in traditional Jewish sources for aborting a foetus based on the foetus' health because it was not possible to know the status of the foetus' health before the advent of modern medical technology. As a result, some religious leaders have ruled that all genetic screening is impermissible because it may lead individuals to abort. Most rabbis have adopted a different approach by arguing that until recently it was not possible to know anything about the health of a foetus, and this new medical knowledge should establish the foetus' health as a separate consideration (Dorff 1996). While this does not resolve the question of under what circumstances a foetus' health justifies abortion, it allows the possibility of abortion. Most Judaic rulings on the permissibility of abortion stem from decisions made in relation to prenatal screening for Tay-Sachs. Rulings will differ by rabbi, and generally each pregnancy is considered on a case by case basis. Jewish attitudes towards genetic screening and abortion are generally open to change whenever new necessities arise or circumstances change (Prainsack and Firestine 2006). All rabbis appear to agree that testing for Tay-Sachs with the ultimate aim of preventing the birth of affected children is desirable, and many current rabbis agree that if a child has already been conceived and it is known that the child will suffer from Tay-Sachs, an abortion is permissible (Rosner 2001). For the ultra-Orthodox, abortion remains generally impermissible – hence the success of Dor Yeshorim which enables couples to avoid abortion. More liberal movements, such as Reform Judaism in the UK, state:

> There is no definitive ruling within Reform on abortion, but there is a strong tendency to favour the liberal viewpoints of Jewish tradition; abortion is allowed in various circumstances where facilities are available for it to be carried out legally and safely. The right of an adult woman to make decisions about her own life and to have sovereignty over her own body are additional factors to be considered. Some Rabbis extend the principle of mental anguish and regard abortion as permissible.
>
> (Movement for Reform Judaism UK 2011)

The connection between Jewish theological beliefs and every day practice is not straightforward, especially given the increasing number of secular or non-practising Jews. As Dorff (1996) points out, most Jews engage in abortion indiscriminately regardless of Jewish theological opinion on abortion. Most of the individuals interviewed during this research were secular and not concerned with Jewish theological views in relation to genetic testing or screening. However, Jewish theology provides an important background because, unlike in other religions, abortion and genetic screening are permissible within Judaism and health is an important priority. These views have underpinned the creation and endorsement of screening programmes specifically for Ashkenazi

Jews by members of various Jewish communities and organizations. This has in turn filtered down to many Jews whether they are theologically observant or not, as evidenced by the fact that almost every individual I encountered was familiar with Tay-Sachs and genetic screening. However, there is more than just Jewish theology at work.

In addition to Jewish theological beliefs, specific cultural and political narratives 'construct biotechnology as crucial for the continuity of Jewish existence' (Prainsack and Firestine 2006: 33). Prainsack and Firestine's (2006) research in Israel found an overwhelmingly positive attitude towards science and technologies, including those that are controversial elsewhere such as reproductive cloning and pre-implantation genetic diagnosis (PGD). The Zionist movement embraced science and technology as crucial tools to maintain the Israeli collective and enable the existence of a Jewish state in the Middle East by transforming the barren desert into fertile land (Prainsack 2007: 88). The first president of the state of Israel, Chaim Weizmann, who was also a scientist, envisaged science as a 'tool to build a new Jewish culture that combines Jewish traditions of 4,000 years with Western progress' (quoted in Prainsack and Firestine 2006: 40). Biotechnologies such as genetic testing and screening, in vitro fertilization (IVF), reproductive cloning and PGD offer the potential to improve, foster and create life for a population continually faced with demographic threats. The Jewish population is in steady decline and maintaining a Jewish population in Israel is crucial to maintaining a Jewish state. Surrounded by Arab neighbours and embroiled in political conflicts, it is essential that Jews maintain the collective body (Prainsack and Firestine 2006: 40). The Holocaust is also an important factor. The loss of six million Jews, and the reproductive consequences in terms of population size, make a high birth rate of healthy Jewish babies especially important (Kahn 2000, Prainsack and Firestine 2006). According to Zertal (2000), the Holocaust has made remembering victims and survivors a universal moral obligation, and the notion of 'never forget' is very often repeated in relation to the Holocaust.

Even outside of Israel, the Holocaust, threats to the survival of the state of Israel, increasing secularization, rising rates of intermarriage and low birth rates have made Jewish survival, reproduction and maintaining future generations particularly important for some Jews. Emma believed that Jewish support for genetics was a direct result of this concern with survival. Her father was born in Germany and had escaped Nazi persecution by taking a transfer with his company to the UK in the late 1930s. Unfortunately he lost all of his immediate family and extended relatives in the Holocaust. Rather than make Emma concerned about genetics, the loss of her father's family reinforced the importance of Jewish survival. Throughout our interview, Emma made numerous references to the miracle that Jews had survived the Holocaust, the importance of maintaining future generations and her own concerns that her daughter had married someone who was not Jewish and the implications for their children's upbringing. In Emma's opinion, knowledge about genetics and health could only be beneficial for Jews, and she cited Dor

Yeshorim as an absolutely 'brilliant and ingenious' example of putting genetic knowledge to good use. Genetic screening appears to offer a way to ensure the continued birth of healthy Jewish children or to keep the population healthy without requiring out-marriage, and this fits well with concerns about Jewish survival. As Cowan (2008) notes, the pronatalist nature of Tay-Sachs screening programmes that permits Jews to continue to produce healthy offspring, especially in the aftermath of the Holocaust, is critical.

Conclusion

Tay-Sachs screening and education programmes, as well as the research that led to the discovery of a carrier test, were instigated, supported and carried out by Ashkenazi Jews. It is unsurprising that they are considered to be unique in their support and endorsement of genetic research and screening (Kronn et al. 1998, Lehman et al. 2002, Levin 2003, Rapp 2000). Ashkenazi Jewish involvement in Tay-Sachs research and screening is undoubtedly a form of biosociality (Rabinow 1996) that pre-dates Rabinow's use of the term to refer to new genetic developments occurring in the 1990s. Why did Ashkenazi Jews take such an active interest in genetic medicine, and conversely why did medical genetics focus so heavily on Ashkenazi Jews? This is not a straight-forward causal relationship but rather one that is mutually constitutive and therefore particularly ripe for being thought of as co-production (Jasanoff 2004). Co-productionist accounts make a strong case against linear, unidirectional causal explanations for complex social phenomena; rather, in this type of account, science and society are co produced, each underwriting the other's existence (Jasanoff 2004: 17). Ashkenazi Jews have been integrally involved in research and screening programmes, and their advocacy has in turn shaped the development of science, as without their involvement the genetic research would not be possible.

Ashkenazi Jews' increased risk of disease is intricately connected to their historical migration patterns, living conditions and cultural context, what Marks (2008) calls 'biosocial' histories. Biological and social histories are interweaved with one another and cannot be disentangled. As a result genetic disease can easily become linked with Jewish history and suffering, and in turn genetic medicine can become a mechanism to address culturally specific issues such as the survival of future generations. Ashkenazi Jews' representation in research is therefore the result of both their increased incidence of genetic disease and also a unique cultural context that has encouraged them to advocate and participate in research. While researchers may have particular interests in Ashkenazi Jews, Ashkenazi Jews have also influenced the research and clinical agenda in many ways.

Specific cultural factors, such as Jewish theology and historical and political context, have also influenced the advocacy and support of Ashkenazi Jews for genetic medicine. The Jewish theological emphasis on health, the permissibility of abortion in certain circumstances, the loss of six million Jews during the

Holocaust, threats to the survival of Israel and a decreasing population all contribute to the success of Tay-Sachs screening. In addition screening was 'community based' (Cowan 2008: 147) and almost all those involved, from the researchers and funders to the educators and volunteers, were Jewish, and most were motivated by personal experience of this traumatic and painful disease and a desire to reduce the suffering it caused. Edelson (1997) points out that exploring the ways in which a disease is 'framed' is a useful approach to examining the acceptance of Tay-Sachs screening by the Ashkenazi Jewish population. From the beginning the community has been 'deeply involved in defining the nature and meaning of Tay-Sachs disease' as one of personal and family tragedy to be avoided if possible (Edelson 1997: 131).

Vulnerability to the potential negative consequences of genetic research and screening programmes will vary for different groups, depending on their social, economic and political power (Duster 1990). Duster (1990) explicitly attributes the reasons for the success of Tay-Sachs programmes, in contrast to those for sickle cell, to the educational and economic position of Ashkenazi Jews as opposed to African Americans. According to Duster (1990), Jews felt sufficiently in control of the politics of screening programmes to allay any potential suspicions. It is important that Jews were involved in the research and development of Tay-Sachs screening, whereas a mandatory sickle cell screening programme was imposed on African Americans by the primarily White government. However, Duster's analysis appears slightly one dimensional and itself reverts to a particular stereotype of Jews as economically and educationally advantaged. Duster emphasizes economic position while ignoring other factors such as Jewish theology, history, concerns with survival, and cultural and political context, all of which have created an environment that is conducive to support for genetic research and screening programmes and help to explain why Ashkenazi Jews are involved in and supportive of genetic medicine.

While there are a variety of factors that contribute to Jewish advocacy of and involvement in genetic screening programmes, it is still difficult to understand how these cultural meta-narratives are enacted on the individual level. In discussing the links between Zionism, the pronatalist Israeli state and women's supportive and uncritical attitudes towards genetic technologies in Israel, Prainsack is careful to point out that this complex nuanced relationship must not be seen in a 'crude' way or as being the result of simple top-down forces (Prainsack 2006: 190). Rather, Prainsack (2006) draws upon Foucault's (1988) technologies of the self to help explain the links. Foucault's (1988: 11) 'technologies of the self' are the practices by which a subject constitutes him- or herself, but these are not practices that the subject devises by him- or herself; rather, they are 'patterns he finds in his culture and which are proposed, suggested and imposed on him by his culture, his society, and his social group'. According to Prainsack (2006: 189), our individual truths are closely connected to the truths or dominant narratives in our society and political and religious 'storylines' can be internalized by individuals.

Much of this chapter has focused on the history of Jewish involvement with genetics and genetic screening programmes. The following chapter turns to the BRCA genes and genetic breast cancer and explores some continuities with Tay-Sachs screening and research, as well as some of the unintended and double-edged consequences resulting from Ashkenazi Jews' early participation in Tay-Sachs screening.

2 The 'Ashkenazi BRCA mutations'

> Jews have travelled a brutal path and repeatedly paid for their continued existence in blood.
>
> (Goldstein 2008: 87)

The history of Jewish involvement with genetic research and screening programmes for Tay-Sachs described in the previous chapter highlighted the role of Ashkenazi Jews as advocates for research and screening programmes, and the culturally specific reasons that contribute to this proactive and supportive attitude. In this chapter I turn to the BRCA genes and in particular draw out some of the continuities and similarities between the developments in BRCA genetic medicine and those of Tay-Sachs. Two recurring themes, the association of BRCA mutations with Jewish history and suffering and the continued role of Ashkenazi Jews as advocates for research and screening, will become evident. The double-edged consequences of participating in research are also examined.

Links with Jewish history

As we have seen, the increased incidence of Tay-Sachs is a result of Jewish historical migration and reproductive patterns and isolation in the ghettos of Eastern Europe. Similar associations with Jewish history and suffering have been made for the Ashkenazi BRCA founder mutations. Population geneticists have dated the three Ashkenazi founder mutations, and each is correlated with a specific event and time point in Jewish history (Neuhausen et al. 1998, Risch et al. 2003, Slatkin 2004). The first mutation (185delAG on BRCA1) is estimated to be between 2,000 and 2,500 years old and is believed to have originated in the Middle East prior to the first important founder event in Ashkenazi Jewish history, when Jews left the Middle East and settled in Europe following the destruction of the Second Temple in around 70 CE (Slatkin 2004). The fact that the mutation is also found in other groups, such as Iraqi Jews, supports the existence of the mutation prior to the divergence of different groups of Jews out of the Middle East and into various Diasporas (Bar-Sade 1998). The second mutation (6174delT on BRCA2) is estimated to be about 700 years old and is believed to have arisen in Eastern Europe as most Jews were settled there at this time. It is associated with a second important founder event – the severe persecution of the Jews during the Crusades and the Black Death, both of which led to an extreme population reduction or bottleneck (Slatkin 2004). Prior to the Crusades in 1096 CE, Jewish populations in Germany, France and England thrived and are estimated to have numbered 100,000. However, during the Crusades attacks on Jews and the destruction of Jewish communities (culminating in their expulsion from England, France and Germany) meant that the population had severely declined by around 1300 CE. The Black Death in 1347/8 led to further population decline, with mortality estimated to have been as high as 50 per cent. This mortality was exacerbated by beliefs that Jews were responsible for spreading the Black Death, leading to further attacks and murders (Slatkin 2004). By 1500 CE Jews in Eastern Europe numbered approximately 10,000 to 20,000 and a period of sustained population growth between the sixteenth and nineteenth centuries followed.

The third mutation (5382insC on BRCA1) is estimated to be about 1,500 to 1,800 years old but only to have entered the Ashkenazi Jewish population approximately 400 years ago. This mutation is associated with a third founder event due to the Cossack massacres in 1648, which resulted in the 'total destruction of many Jewish communities' and the death of at least 25 per cent of the population (Risch et al. 1995: 157). How did this mutation, which arose elsewhere, enter the Ashkenazi Jewish population 400 years ago? According to one Jewish breast surgeon I worked with, the mutation may have spread as a result of rapes during pogroms, leading him to describe it as 'another tragic event in Jewish history' and 'component in the repertoire of humiliations experienced in the Jewish ghettos of the Pale of Settlement between the 13th and 19th centuries' (Report of the Anglo-Israeli workshop on the genetic risk of breast cancer, 2006: 4). Of course rape is not the only mechanism by which genes can be transferred across groups, and this surgeon's comment demonstrates how specific aspects of Ashkenazi Jewish historical suffering are invoked to explain hereditary disease-causing mutations. In contrast, Hamel et al. (2011: 305) claim that the rapid expansion of Jews in Eastern Europe from the sixteenth century 'significantly improved the odds of admixture' between Jews and non-Jews, even for an otherwise relatively genetically isolated group. Admixture refers to reproduction across groups and is a more neutral way of explaining how and why the mutation spread between Jews and non-Jews during this time. Despite being known as 'Ashkenazi founder mutations', two of the three mutations can be found in other Jewish and non-Jewish populations, raising questions about why they continue to be designated 'Ashkenazi' at all.

Between 2004 and 2010, I worked on an international chemotherapy clinical trial for BRCA mutation carriers with metastatic breast cancer in London, England. The trial was especially important because it was the first attempt to tailor treatment specifically for BRCA mutation carriers, who until that point were treated with the same drug therapies as all other breast cancer patients. There was increasing evidence that specific characteristics of BRCA tumours made them more sensitive and responsive to particular treatments, such as platinum-based chemotherapy, which might therefore be more effective in BRCA mutation carriers (Balmaña et al. 2011). From the outset of the clinical trial, recruiting Ashkenazi Jewish women was considered crucial to reaching the required number of study subjects because of their high incidence of founder mutations. Articles were written in the *Jewish Chronicle* newspaper to promote the trial (Fletcher 2007, Symons 2006) and, most significantly, separate funding was sought and granted to open the trial in Israel, where it was hoped many eligible women would be recruited.[1] One of the collaborating clinicians for this project, who is Jewish himself, regularly visited Israel to promote and encourage what was called the 'Anglo-Israeli Collaboration'. He is an eminent breast surgeon who is well respected and known in the breast cancer clinical world. In April 2006 English and Israeli scientists and clinicians met at a workshop in Israel to discuss this particular trial and other potential genetic breast cancer research collaborations. The way in which the BRCA mutations create links to Jewish history and suffering was particularly evident in the report prepared following the meeting, which described it as:

> A journey through the land of Israel, the history of the Jewish people, our genealogy and genetic anthropology, as well as a consideration of the mutations that pre-dispose to breast cancer ... when you look at the individual genes you see how the history of the Jewish people has been reflected, once again, on the molecular level.
>
> (Report of the Anglo-Israeli workshop on the genetic
> risk of breast cancer 2006)

Just like Tay-Sachs, the BRCA founder mutations are directly related to the Jewish ancestral past and the history of Jewish suffering, which further illustrates how genetic disease can become entangled with Jewish identity (Wailoo and Pemberton 2006). Montoya (2007) uses the term 'bioethnic conscription' to describe the ways in which 'social identities and life conditions of DNA donors are grafted onto the biological explanations of disease causality' (2007: 94). He describes DNA collection from Mexicans in the US, as well as discussions about the genetics of Haitians, and argues that the social histories of these populations, including slavery, colonialism, genocide and other factors, play a significant role in deciding their genetic utility.

Disease as punishment

Some of the women interviewed did associate their genetic risk of breast cancer with Jewish history, and particularly Jewish suffering. Rachel was a secular unmarried woman in her late forties who had been born in the United States but had lived in London for nearly 25 years. She had left her job in adult education and was in the process of considering a career change and possibly becoming an art teacher. Rachel had attended the clinic for information and advice about genetic testing, following a referral from her general practitioner. Her sister was a BRCA1 mutation carrier who had developed breast cancer at 51 years old, although Rachel had not yet decided if she wanted to undergo testing. Rachel's family history was on her paternal side, where her aunt who had breast cancer was also a known BRCA mutation carrier. Rachel's great-grandparents were from Eastern Europe but the following generations in her family had all been born in the United States. Rachel described her connection to Eastern Europe as being 'far back' but that the mutations drew her back in history despite this distance:

> But funny how history can then be passed down and so many years later ... I mean I'm thinking about my sister 'cuz she's not married to a Jew and so the girls aren't even, they're like half Jewish ... it doesn't matter what you've chosen it's still in your genes from way back, it's strange.

Genes are an inescapable link to the Jewish past and, despite the fact that Rachel's sister had married someone non-Jewish, this did not decrease the risk of her daughters inheriting the mutations (a topic that will be returned to in chapter six). During our interview Rachel had asked me about why these mutations had come about and we discussed the founder mutations, which she related to the history of oppression:

> Are you being punished for your behaviour? Because that's coming from a place of people who have been oppressed, isn't it? Or excluded or whatever and then it's just strange then, yeah. I mean it kind of makes sense why that would happen.

Rachel made a comparison to one of her homosexual friends who was screened annually for HIV and felt that HIV could seem like a punishment for being gay, an identity that he experienced as marginalizing and oppressive.

Susan was a 39-year-old British married mother of two who was religiously observant. She was finishing a professional graduate degree and was one of three relatives in the family that I interviewed (along with her sister Anna and first cousin Jennifer). Susan had a strong family history of breast cancer and had lost her mother to the disease when she was 20. She had undergone genetic testing and was due to receive her results the day after our interview. Susan also referred to the Ashkenazi founder mutations in relation to Jewish history and as a possible punishment:

SUSAN: The genes situation came from historically a long time ago ... it's just a real mystery ... I really don't get it, *why us* type of thing? [emphasis added]

JM: Do you ever feel like that?

SUSAN: Yeah! But when I'm worrying about things it's more localized and personal like why my mother, you know, why us? Not 'the people', although I am part of a people but you know all the tribes are joined up so I mean I don't really think in terms of historically my people.

Susan related the mutations to her 'people' and their history; however, she acknowledged that she experienced her risk in a more personal way in relation to her own mother and family rather than to the Jewish people as a whole.

I was repeatedly told variations of a story, a type of Jewish genetic disease legend, which involves a non-Jewish individual of some importance, stature or wealth who marries and then gives birth to a child with Tay-Sachs. The birth of the child with Tay-Sachs is proof that this individual is actually Jewish, but their identity had been suppressed or deliberately hidden for some reason. Despite the fact that both parents must be carriers of the Tay-Sachs mutation for a child to be born with the disease, the story is used to show that genetic disease can reveal previously unknown or hidden Jewish identity. As Neulander (2006) notes, legends always take place in a historical time and are stories involving a historical person, place or event but about something that cannot be secured or verified in history. David was a dentist and medical researcher in his mid-fifties with no family history of disease. He was married and had two children. He was born and raised in South Africa, although he had lived in London for over 35 years. During our interview, he recounted his variation of the story:

> There was a very, very auspicious family in South Africa, the X family, and the Xs converted to Christianity for all sorts of reasons. And nice Christian family marry another Christian girl and guess what? Out comes Tay-Sachs, and of course all of our Orthodox friends said: 'You see divine retribution. You want to convert to Christianity? You want to marry a Christian? That is what you get. It comes back to haunt you. You can't get rid of it.'

David then remembered that Tay-Sachs was recessive, and noted that both individuals would have to be carriers for the child to be born with Tay-Sachs: 'So it has to be both the male and the female … *live with your guilt* now' (emphasis added).

David's story implies not only that the existence of genetic disease can reveal a previous hidden Jewish identity, but that it may even be a punishment for marrying out or trying to conceal your Jewish identity – a form of 'divine retribution'. David suggests that individuals should feel guilty for passing on genetic mutations or trying to hide their Jewishness and that, despite efforts to hide one's identity, 'Jewish genes' will always prevail. I heard similar stories about the BRCA genes. One genetic counsellor told me that sometimes they find the 'Ashkenazi mutations' in families who do not think they are Jewish. I enquired whether this actually indicates that a family is really Jewish given that some of these mutations are present in non-Jewish Eastern European individuals. She informed me that it just shows you how 'somewhere back there genes got mixed in', and that she usually chose not to inform the family that the mutation was specifically a Jewish one.

Neulander's (2006) research in New Mexico with non-Jewish individuals found to carry supposedly 'Jewish' genetic diseases or mutations shows how genetic disease can be used to infer 'secret' or 'crypto-Jewish' descent from ancestral Jews. These claims often serve a broader purpose of asserting an overvalued line of White ancestral descent and restoring 'prestige lineage'. Neulander (2006) argues that the use of the label 'Jewish' to determine who is at risk of genetic disease has paved the way for the popular use of heritable diseases to determine who is a Jew. This 'disease-based Judaism' (Neulander 2006: 389) is in fact a failure to differentiate between heritable characteristics acquired through DNA and cultural characteristics widely attributed to Jews which are only acquired through learning. Neulander (2006) argues strongly against genetically labelling faith-based communities and instead proposes that diseases are identified in terms of geographical origins, such as Eastern Europe rather than Ashkenazi Jewish, since every heritable disease will have a founder who can be located in time and place.

Neulander (2006) also cautions that scientists who are charged with identifying patterns within the human genome are not trained to recognize the negative scientific and social consequences of labelling disease according to non-heritable and essentially untestable cultural characteristics (Neulander 2006: 395). A scientific study by Weitzel et al. (2005) to determine the frequency of BRCA mutations among Hispanic American women living in Los Angeles found a high number of the Ashkenazi founder mutations in the sample. This led them to conclude that these 'apparently non-Jewish' families must have been descended from the Spanish Jews, known as conversos, who hid their identities during periods of anti-Semitism in Spain from the twelfth to sixteenth centuries (Weitzel et al. 2005: 1669). Rather than raising doubts about whether the mutations are specific to Ashkenazi Jews, the researchers' conclusion reinforces the notion of 'Jewish genes'. Finkler (2001: 248) claims that DNA remembers what has long been forgotten and that 'people cannot invent or appropriate ancestors, because a DNA test will reveal the truth'. The 'relentless transmission' of DNA from generation to generation creates continuity and connections with not only present but also past relations (Finkler 2001: 248). For both professionals working in medical genetics and lay Jewish individuals, mutations in the BRCA genes can be used to infer Jewish origins, as evidence of the history of oppression and suffering of the Jews, and even as a possible punishment.

The ability of genetic research to reveal 'Jewish genes' and reiterate identity is further illustrated by two population genetic studies that received much media and popular attention. The Cohen modal haplotype is a genetic marker found on the Y chromosome that has been used to identify Jews who are supposedly descended from ancient Jewish Cohanim priests (Goldstein 2008,

Thomas et al. 2000). The Cohanim were a biblical priestly class of Jewish men who traced their roots back to Aaron, the brother of Moses. Being a Cohen priest was passed down from father to son and the surname Cohen is still common today. The Y chromosome is carried only by men (in contrast, women carry two X chromosomes) and is therefore exclusively passed from father to son. As opposed to the other 22 chromosomes, it does not recombine with other DNA during reproduction and so is passed from father to son relatively intact without any changes in the sequence of DNA, making it an effective way to trace paternal lineage. Researchers compared the Y chromosome of various Jewish groups to that of non-Jews and discovered there was a 'Cohen modal haplotype' (a set of polymorphisms that occurs more often) found on the Y chromosome of some Jewish men who identify themselves as Cohens.[2] Carrying the Cohen modal haplotype has been used to confirm or 'prove' the Jewish origins of various groups in Asia and Africa. For example, the Lemba are a Black South African tribe who claim to be descendants of one of the lost tribes of Israel. They have some traditions, such as circumcision, dietary laws and rituals related to conversion, that are similar to those of Judaism. Thomas et al. (2000) discovered that some of the Lemba carried the Cohen modal haplotype and this was used as evidence that they were likely descended from Jews in ancient Israel, as their oral history suggests. Another group of Jews in Ethiopia who claim also to be descended from Jews in ancient Israel were tested and did not carry the haplotype, and this was taken as proof that they were not Jewish (Azoulay 2003). Private companies now offer testing for the Cohen modal haplotype to Jews across the world to determine if they are descendants of this biblical priestly class of Jews.

The second genetic study relates to mitochondrial DNA (Behar et al. 2006). Mitochondrial DNA is passed only from mothers to children (both sons and daughters) and, like the Y chromosome, it does not recombine with other DNA and is therefore a useful way of tracing maternal lineage. In this particular study, the mitochondrial DNA of Ashkenazi and non-Ashkenazi Jews was compared and it was concluded that nearly half of the world's Ashkenazi Jewish population can be traced to four founding women who existed in Europe within the last 2,000 years (Behar et al. 2006). Both these population genetic studies were widely reported in the international media, including ABC news, MSNBC, *USA Today* and the *New York Times*, and PBS made a documentary about the Cohen modal haplotype research (Gessen 2008). In November 2006 the London Jewish Cultural Centre offered an entire three-week course devoted to the Cohen research, entitled 'The Lost Jews of Africa'.

Mitochondrial DNA and Y chromosome studies generate knowledge about ancestry and create links between Ashkenazi Jews in the present and their biological ancestors, and they reiterate the descent of Jews from a common and fairly homogeneous ancestral group (Kahn 2005). Brodwin (2002) claims these studies privilege genetics in determining identity above other claims such as oral history, written documentation, cultural practices and inner convictions, ignoring the social ways in which identity is constructed. One of the lead scientists of the Cohen modal haplotype research acknowledges that genetics forms only one small part of a much larger story that includes history, texts, culture, archaeology and many other areas of enquiry (Goldstein 2008). Another of the contributing researchers to the Cohen modal haplotype research explained that genetic identity is just one of many ways in which Jewish identity is formed but acknowledged that it is potentially confusing to have studies which seem to imply that being Jewish is genetic (personal communication). Brodwin (2002) warns that being a carrier of the Cohen modal haplotype could be used in order to make citizenship claims to Israel, although this has not yet occurred. As Rose (2007) astutely notes, the issue at stake is not discrimination but damage to identity because these studies have the potential to undermine or corroborate a group's creation story or communal narrative and to challenge or transform how individuals and groups come to understand their affinities and distinctions. In the case of Ashkenazi Jews, these studies corroborate a communal narrative, although Azoulay (2006) is highly critical of such studies and argues that the precondition of a 'Cohen gene' is supposed common ancestry, which ignores the explicitly social ways in which identity is constructed.

The previous section has concentrated on the connections between genetics, disease-causing mutations, and Jewish history and suffering, something that was also evident in relation to Tay-Sachs. The following section turns to the second similarity with Tay-Sachs, that of Jewish advocacy for BRCA research and testing. Once again, the correlation of genetic breast cancer with specific aspects of Jewish history means that it can easily become entangled with Jewish preservation and survival, another factor that advocacy groups have focused on.

Biosocial coalitions and BRCA advocacy

This section describes the biosocial coalitions and genetic alliances that have been formed by Ashkenazi Jewish women at risk of genetic breast cancer (see also Rabinow 1996, Raz 2010, Rose 2007, Taussig et al. 2003). Taussig et al.'s (2003) study of the US advocacy organization Little People of America (representing people of short stature or dwarves) describes the cooperative relationship between those born with dwarfism and medical and genetic researchers as a 'biosocial coalition'. The gene for achondroplasia (dwarfism) was discovered in 1994 as a result of long-term work and the collection of research samples from patients all over the world whose tissue was held in a registry. Patient advocates belonging to the Little People of America (LPA) contributed to 'laboratory and clinical knowledge through their tissue samples in countless experimental and diagnostic contexts, and through the emotional knowledge that families living with genetically different members accumulate' (Taussig et al. 2003: 58). Such biosocial coalitions may be double-edged, as was the case with the discovery of the gene for achondroplasia which introduced the possibility of screening for, and possibly eliminating, those born with the disease, something not all members of the LPA supported.

The samples donated by Ashkenazi Jews taking part in Tay-Sachs screening programmes had direct implications for the discovery of the Ashkenazi BRCA mutations and provide an example of how participating in genetic research can result in both gifts and poisons (Taussig et al. 2003, Wailoo and Pemberton 2006). The identification of the first Ashkenazi founder mutation on BRCA1 was derived from a set of approximately 700 Tay-Sachs samples that had been stored since the 1970s. Tay-Sachs screening brought thousands of Ashkenazi Jews into clinics where their blood samples were not only tested for Tay-Sachs but often stored for future genetic research. The 'unexpected research payoff' (Kahn 2005: 8) was the availability of stored blood samples that were subsequently used for other research studies. Whether or not individuals consented to this future research remains an ethically unresolved issue (Rothenberg 1997). The US National Institute for Health (NIH), with the support of Jewish community leaders in the Washington area, then conducted a follow-up study on over 5,000 Ashkenazi men and women who willingly donated additional samples to determine the frequency of this BRCA mutation (Dorff 1997, Rothenberg 1997). Members of various Jewish organizations approved the protocol, consent form and recruitment procedures for the study and Jewish leaders actively encouraged people to participate, while many synagogues and Jewish community centres served as study sites (Rothenberg 1997, Struewing et al. 1997).

Dor Yeshorim has also played a significant role in research and discoveries related to other 'Jewish genetic diseases', particularly by sharing samples with genetic researchers, which has helped to validate the genetic mutations that cause Canavan disease, Gaucher type1 and Fanconi anaemia. Dor Yeshorim has also provided financial support to selected researchers and facilitated patient recruitment to research studies (Prainsack and Siegal 2006). According to the founder of Dor Yeshorim, Rabbi Ekstein, this 'synergy' between prevention of disease and research is a 'valuable outcome of the firm base of trust and participation that Dor Yeshorim has established in its community' (Ekstein and Katzenstein 2001: 308). For Raz (2010), the addition of other genetic recessive diseases to Dor Yeshorim, including some that are not fatal, have variable severity and may be treatable (such as Gaucher's disease), raises serious ethical concerns.

As a result of these 'biosocial coalitions' (Taussig et al. 2003), new information about the Ashkenazi population has continued to emerge based on the samples, and in addition to this there has been a tendency to categorize all findings as 'Jewish diseases' despite the fact that the same diseases or mutations may exist in other populations who have just not yet been studied (Wailoo and Pemberton 2006). The research has become self-perpetuating as investigations continue to build upon this pre-existing large body of literature and samples (Birenbaum Carmeli 2004). The fact that Jews may simply come to the attention of scientists and doctors more often, for example because of their proximity to large urban clinical and research centres, is known as 'ascertainment bias' (Goldstein 2008). Jews' historical involvement in research has led to an ascertainment bias and may not actually represent a greater burden of disease than is present in other populations. This illustrates the way in which knowledge of genetic disease among specific groups is a reflection not only of their actual risk but also of the availability of samples and a positive participatory attitude towards research and medicine, and is yet another way in which science and society are co-produced (Jasanoff 2004).

Raz (2010: 115) describes genetic alliances as 'social networks of individuals genetically at risk', which can include online support networks, disease-specific support groups, and alliances of support groups. Genetic alliances help patients with the same condition become aware of the similarity of their individual experiences and develop a collective 'biosocial' awareness. Support groups for patients can have several functions, including participation in public policy decision-making with health professional and industry leaders, empowering individuals at risk to make informed, autonomous decisions about the utilization of genetic services, campaigning for rights and combating stigma, contributing to the advancement of genetic research, and communicating the needs of those living with disease to health care professionals. These groups can exert significant pressure for research to be carried out that can identify genetic tests, screening tests and treatments for the families or communities affected (Rose 2007). The Genetic Alliance is a network comprising over 1,000 disease-specific advocacy organizations, as well as universities, private companies, government agencies and public policy organizations, and is the world's leading non-profit health advocacy organization committed to transforming health through genetics. Their mission is to bring together diverse stakeholders to promote novel partnerships in advocacy, integrate individual family and community perspectives to improve health systems, and to revolutionize access to information to enable research and individualized decision-making.[3]

There are four genetic breast cancer advocacy organizations within the Genetic Alliance, two of which are devoted solely to Ashkenazi Jewish women – JACOB and Sharsheret. Jews against Cancers of the Breast (JACOB) International is dedicated to helping Ashkenazi Jewish women learn more about their increased risk of genetic breast cancer. Their goal is not only to educate Ashkenazi women but also to encourage all women (not just those at high risk) to seek genetic testing in order to fulfil their mission of breaking the cycle of hereditary breast and ovarian cancer. According to their website:

> Our organization is for this generation and all that follows in its footsteps. We can give a gift of a longer life to someone who carries this mutation – a gift that we hope can be passed down to other generations.
>
> (JACOB 2011)

The organization was founded by Lori, an Ashkenazi Jewish woman who was diagnosed with breast cancer at the age of 47. After her diagnosis, she was found to be a BRCA1 mutation carrier and her two sisters then underwent testing as well. Following Lori's death, the organization was taken over by her husband and two surviving sisters. In describing Lori, and why the organization is so important, the website states:

> Just imagine if Lori's doctor, the Jewish community, our family or a friend had educated us on the benefits of genetic testing. Lori could have had a prophylactic mastectomy and hysterectomy, avoided chemotherapy and would be alive today. But then again, perhaps this was Lori's path and purpose to EDUCATE you so that this is not your story and not the story of any future generations. *We will break the cycle of L'dor Vador* when it comes to hereditary breast and ovarian cancer ... *May we, as a Jewish people, go from strength to greater strength!!!*
>
> (JACOB 2011, emphasis added)

'L'dor vador' is Hebrew for 'from generation to generation' and the website explicitly associates being tested for the Ashkenazi BRCA founder mutations with the health of all future Jews. The website has a section containing Hebrew prayers devoted to healing and is available in Hebrew, Spanish, Portuguese, Russian and French. The advisory board consists of genetic counsellors, clinicians, representatives from Myriad, rabbis and other Jewish religious leaders and organizations.

Sharsheret (Hebrew for 'chain') is an American non-profit organization of Jewish breast cancer survivors that was founded in 2001. Sharsheret supports young Jewish women and their families facing breast cancer and acknowledges the 'unique concerns' of Jewish women particularly by putting them in contact with one another and offering various support programmes. Its mission is to provide a community of support to women diagnosed with breast cancer or at increased genetic risk by fostering culturally relevant individualized connections with networks of peers, health professionals and related resources. Since its founding, it has responded to more than 19,000 breast cancer enquiries, and it offers peer support and educational programmes nationwide.

While JACOB is more explicit in its mission to promote genetic testing, both organizations focus on the role of genetics and testing as ways to prevent breast cancer and possibly protect future generations, with strong discourses of hope and survival (see also Raz 2010). Gilman's (2003) analysis of support websites for families of children with other 'Jewish genetic diseases' has shown the ways in which a disease can become a Jewish disease and all its sufferers part of an extended and interrelated family linked by their experience of shared disease. JACOB's website explains the Ashkenazi mutations as follows:

> It is believed that these mutations can be traced back hundreds of years to their common ancestors, or founders. As the result of numerous inter-marriages among Jews, all of today's Ashkenazi Jews are descended from a very small group of Jews who lived in Eastern Europe 500 years ago.

These 'founding Ashkenazis' carried the particular BRCA1 and BRCA2 gene mutations which were subsequently passed on to their descendants.

(JACOB 2011)

Most BRCA advocacy has primarily occurred in the United States; there are no specific BRCA advocacy or support organizations for Ashkenazi Jewish women in the UK. This may partially be a reflection of the differences in the 'architecture of genetic testing' (Parthasarathy 2007) between the US and UK. Parthasarathy (2007) has shown how the differing national, social and political contexts of the UK and US affected the way in which BRCA testing systems developed, with the health systems being particularly influential. Private commercial testing via Myriad has dominated the US market-based and consumer-driven approach (also described in the introduction) and this has resulted in inequitable access to testing in the US health care system (see Mozersky and Joseph 2010). In the UK, efforts have focused on centralized and integrated clinical and laboratory services, with the National Health Service acting as gatekeeper for the test, which is offered (free of charge) to those who meet the high-risk criteria set by the National Institute for Health and Clinical Excellence (NICE 2005).

Regardless of where they originate, advocacy efforts drive forward research and knowledge with international implications. Patient and advocacy groups, such as JACOB and Sharsheret, are self-defined activist communities mobilized by the hope of a cure that campaign energetically for research (Rose 2007: 174). The *Jewish Chronicle* newspaper carried an article in 2006 about a woman who developed breast cancer and, once 'alerted to the greater risks faced by Ashkenazi women', received advocacy training from a large UK breast cancer charity and now addresses synagogues and Jewish groups throughout London (Symons 2006). For Ashkenazi Jews, the increased risk of genetic breast cancer is an opportunity to mobilize and take action to prevent disease for the entire 'community' (especially because it is associated with Jewish history and future generations). This is further illustrated by the development of BRCA population screening programmes, which are discussed in the following section.

Population screening

From a clinical perspective, population screening has been under discussion for some time in the UK and abroad. Population screening involves screening all consenting Ashkenazi individuals for BRCA mutations, regardless of family or personal history of cancer. It is feasible and cost effective within the Ashkenazi population because of the three known founder mutations that make screening technically simple and rapid (Grann et al. 1999). Yet the psychological and social consequences of this approach remain unknown. The majority of psychosocial studies have drawn on high-risk individuals with family histories, many of whom are already involved in research. High-risk individuals have a pre-existing sense of risk and may be more prepared for a positive test result than those who have no prior experience with, or knowledge of, the disease in question (Durfy et al. 1999, Nelson et al. 2005). It has been shown that a positive test result may cause more distress if it is unexpected (Croyle et al. 1997, Watson et al. 1996). Shkedi-Rafid's (2012) study looking at the implications of BRCA genetic testing among those without family histories in Israel found that while the idea was generally supported by individuals, those with no family history did experience some confusion and vulnerability when they tested positive.

Part of the rationale behind only screening those considered to be at high risk is that the management options available for BRCA1 and BRCA2 mutation carriers are invasive or limited (Grann et al. 1999). Surgical removal of the breasts and ovaries is the only known way to almost entirely eliminate the future risk of breast and ovarian cancer for carriers, although even this option does not completely eliminate risk, and there remains no absolutely reliable method of early diagnosis (Mor and Oberle 2008). The main benefit of population screening is that those who are at increased risk, and would not otherwise have been tested, can take the relevant preventative measures. Neither the guidelines of the American Society for Clinical Oncology (Robson et al. 2010) nor Nelson et al.'s (2005) systematic review of the benefits and harms of general population screening recommend BRCA mutation screening for any population.

Population screening for BRCA is different from that for recessive diseases such as Tay-Sachs because carrying a single copy of a BRCA mutation can cause disease. The BRCA mutations are transmitted in an autosomal dominant fashion so that the offspring of a carrier has a 50 per cent chance of inheriting the mutation from the carrier parent. In contrast, recessive diseases are only manifested when the offspring of two carriers inherits both copies of the mutation because carrying a single copy does not cause disease (as described in chapter one). This is the underlying rationale behind recessive screening programmes, as the identification of carrier status offers a way of preventing disease primarily through prenatal screening, with abortion of the affected foetus (although other options are available). For BRCA mutation carriers, the only way to prevent a child inheriting the mutation is to use in vitro fertilization (IVF) followed by pre-implantation genetic diagnosis (PGD), where embryos are selected for implantation only once they have been tested for the mutation and found to be negative. The first BRCA-free baby was born in December 2008 following PGD performed at University College London.[4] This story was widely covered in the media throughout the world. As in the case of recessive diseases, the use of donor gametes, adoption or deciding not to have children are also possible options. Another difference is that breast cancer is a late onset and treatable disease and not all carriers of BRCA mutations will develop breast or ovarian cancer as the genes are not 100 per cent penetrant. In contrast, Tay-Sachs is always lethal in childhood and no treatment exists.

In the late 1990s questions arose about whether BRCA testing would be added to the Dor Yeshorim screening programme. The founder of Dor Yeshorim, Rabbi Ekstein, publicly stated that testing for BRCA mutations would not become part of Dor Yeshorim because the genes were dominant and screening could not prevent the birth of an affected child, and because breast cancer was a late onset, and not necessarily fatal, disease (Wailoo and Pemberton 2006). This decision followed tensions that had arisen in the ultra-Orthodox community, as some rabbis were concerned that the increasing number of diseases being added to Dor Yeshorim could be harmful and potentially misunderstood to mean that Jews were more ill. Such fears have not hindered the recent development of BRCA population screening programmes in the UK, Canada and Israel, which have the support of local Jewish communities and organizations.

In the UK, a pilot population screening programme began in October 2008. It aims to recruit 10,000 Ashkenazi Jews and, according to the study website, 'to develop a strategy for prediction and prevention of genetic cancer. Over the long term it is hoped this will reduce cancers in the community.'[5] The study has received support from the major Jewish charity in the UK, Jewish Care, as well as the Liberal and Reform Jewish movements, rabbis, other Jewish organizations and a major high-street chemist. As in the UK, it was announced in May 2008 that Jewish women in Ontario, Canada, would be offered a free genetic test for BRCA mutations as part of a research study. Within 10 days of a national Canadian newspaper advertising the study, over 2,100 women had volunteered, illustrating 'considerable interest for genetic testing among Jewish women' (Metcalfe et al. 2009: 1). This study found that 45 per cent of the mutations identified were in women who did not meet the local genetic testing criteria, leading the authors to conclude that genetic testing should be extended to women who do not meet the current criteria (Metcalfe et al. 2009). One female Canadian rabbi claimed that BRCA mutation screening will one day be offered in a similar way to screening for Tay-Sachs because the 'rate of this gene is so high' (Priest 2008). A Canadian newspaper described this study as follows:

> According to research, 40 per cent of today's Ashkenazi Jewish population arose from a group of 4 founding mothers who lived somewhere in Europe within the past 2000 years. With the marvels of science, their female descendants are being offered the opportunity to peek into the genetic version of a crystal ball.
>
> (Priest 2008)

A general population screening study in Israel has recently completed recruitment and found similar results to the Canadian study; that is, mutations were identified in 63 per cent of families that would not have otherwise been considered high risk as they had minimal or no family history of breast or ovarian cancer (Levy-Lahad et al. 2011). Importantly, these Ashkenazi families often had unique pedigrees with a small family size, paternal inheritance or a preponderance of male relatives. Pedigrees may also be affected if many relatives in previous generations were lost in the Holocaust. The Israeli study concludes that population-wide screening of the Ashkenazi population is feasible, cost effective and justified (Levy-Lahad et al. 2011).

Margaret Lock (1998) likens genetic testing for breast cancer to traditional forms of divination, which produce knowledge that is not readily available to ordinary people. According to Lock (1998: 7), current genetic testing permits us to divine our past and to make that heritage – in the form of genes – into omens for the future. The Ashkenazi BRCA mutations divine the Jewish ancestral past and historical events, as we have seen above, while at the same time offering important information about the future health of carriers and their offspring.

Conclusion

This chapter has focused on the continuities between current developments and research related to the Ashkenazi BRCA mutations and the Tay-Sachs research and screening described in chapter one. The first continuity is the association of BRCA mutations with collective Jewish history and suffering. Research has correlated the BRCA founder mutations with specific events and time points in Jewish history and so, as in the case of Tay-Sachs, genetic breast cancer and the mutations that cause it can become intertwined with Jewish suffering and survival (Wailoo and Pemberton 2006). There was evidence that some women interpreted genetic mutations as punishment, and that genetic mutations could even be used to infer Jewish origins. This 'disease-based Judaism' (Neulander 2006) was evident in individual stories and research studies, where the existence of supposedly 'Jewish' mutations was used to confirm or reveal previously unknown Jewish identity. Genetic disease and mutations simultaneously reflect and reiterate Jewish collective history and origins, as do population genetic studies such as the Cohen modal haplotype and mitochondrial DNA studies.

The second continuity between Tay-Sachs and BRCA is evident in Ashkenazi Jewish advocacy for BRCA genetic research, screening and testing. Advocacy groups such as JACOB and Sharsheret promote genetic testing, and population screening programmes for BRCA mutations are under way. These developments have the support of Jewish organizations and/or are initiated by Ashkenazi Jews. For populations who are at risk, finding the biological substrates for disease increases the possibilities of effective intervention in the name of health, and genetic medicine can be seen as allying itself with the demands and concerns of a specific biosocial group, gaining the support of the relevant community bodies and committed physicians, and addressing relevant problems (Rose 2007: 183).

The Environmental Breast Cancer Movement (EBCM) provides an interesting contrast to the relative lack of critical debate among Ashkenazi Jewish advocacy groups about the genetic basis of breast cancer. The EBCM is devoted to challenging biomedical claims about the cause of breast cancer (Zavestoski et al. 2004) and can be thought of as a biosocial collective forged around an active rejection of the ways in which modern biomedicine classifies individuals or their disease (Rabinow 1996). According to the EBCM, the dominant paradigm of breast cancer causation focuses on the genetic and biological explanations for disease, with prevention primarily aimed at the individual level. This biomedical focus neglects the environmental factors that might contribute to disease, as well as possible prevention efforts, and instead places responsibility on individual women, whether through genetics or lifestyle factors. The US advocacy organization Breast Cancer Action (BCA) is devoted to raising awareness about the environmental causes of breast cancer and specifically claims that biological explanations divert attention away from more important causal factors that contribute to breast cancer, including social, political, economic and racial inequalities. BCA advocacy focuses on raising awareness about commercialization, corporate conflicts of interest and diversion of breast cancer research funds. For example, their 'Think Pink' campaign encourages women to boycott pink-ribbon campaigns and the companies that they call 'pinkwashers'. Pinkwashers are organizations or companies that 'claim to care about breast cancer by promoting a pink ribbon product, but at the same time produce, manufacture and/or sell products that are linked to the disease' (Breast Cancer Action 2011). The ways in which research into the genetic causation of breast cancer reiterates specific aspects of shared Jewish history and communal narratives, while genetic testing and screening offer ways to alter the health of future generations, may contribute to the acceptance of and lack of critical debate about genetic explanations (see also Prainsack 2007).

While advocacy and genetic screening can have significant health benefits, such as the identification of those who are at increased risk or a reduction in the number of children born with disease, alongside these benefits participation in research may have unintended consequences, such as becoming over-represented. The continued involvement of and donation of samples by Ashkenazi Jews, beginning with Tay-Sachs screening in the 1970s and continuing today with BRCA research, mean that samples will continue to accumulate, knowledge will build, and as a result diseases will continue to be designated as 'Jewish'. The following chapter further addresses these potential negative consequences of genetic research by exploring whether individuals had concerns about current genetic research.

3 Rethinking the consequences of medical genetic research

The previous chapter demonstrated how the BRCA mutations reiterate connections with Jewish history, including the history of suffering, while advocacy groups that promote testing and population screening programmes offer ways to alter the future health of Jews and potentially eliminate disease. The proactive and participatory relationship between Ashkenazi Jews and genetic medicine has undoubtedly had beneficial consequences, such as the reduction of disease and the availability of carrier screening. However, this involvement has been double-edged and there have been unintended consequences, such as becoming over-represented in research and the discovery of new 'Jewish' diseases simply because samples are available. Concerns have been raised about the implications of genetic knowledge and research for Ashkenazi Jews, and this chapter begins with a discussion of these concerns. Qualitative interview material is used to explore how high-risk women experience their clinical encounters and whether individuals have concerns about being the subjects of genetic research/medicine focused on Ashkenazi Jews. In the final part of the chapter I draw out some implications of these findings, critically reflecting on the dominant thinking about the implications of genetic research for populations and drawing attention to the fact that not all populations are the same, or necessarily vulnerable to the consequences of genetic knowledge in the same ways.

Implications of genetic research for Ashkenazi Jews

The first main criticism regarding genetic research of Ashkenazi Jews is based on historical misuses of genetics and the potential continuities with previous discrimination and anti-Semitism. Anti-Semitism has historically been undergirded by a biological and genetic determinism about supposed biological differences between Jews and non-Jews (Glenn 2010), and this history unsurprisingly dominates concerns about contemporary research. There is a long-standing historical association of European Jews with disease and ill health, and the question of the health of the Jews was raised frequently in many different circles and countries throughout Europe, beginning in medieval times and lasting through the nineteenth century (Gilman 1985: 154). Medical and anthropological societies in Poland, Germany, France and Austria presented reports, papers and statistics about the ill health and predisposition to disease among the Jewish population. The tendency to associate Jews with ill health was often part of other anti-Semitic campaigns or beliefs about the differences and inferiority of the Jews, such as state-imposed confinement to particular areas (Gilman 1985: 151). The association of Jews with illness was also exploited for political purposes. Proponents of the emancipation of Jews argued that their illness was a result of the repression imposed on them by the state or their religious practices such as early marriage. These things were changeable and so was the health of the Jews. In contrast, those who were not in favour of political emancipation argued that Jews were ill by nature regardless of their status, religious practices or context and should not be granted political freedom or equality (Gilman 1985: 152). They were considered naturally degenerate and thus no action needed to be taken to change their conditions.

Most notably, during the Second World War eugenic claims that Jews were 'genetically inferior' contributed to and provided part of the underlying justification for the Holocaust and mass murder of Jews (as well as other groups). They also led many countries to enact very restrictive immigration policies that limited the number of Jews trying to escape from Nazi Germany who were allowed in. Gilman (2003) warns that current genetic findings may lead to a return to the past or result in renewed discrimination, stigmatization or an increase in racism towards Jews. Neulander (2006: 396) claims that it is almost inevitable that classifications of genetic diseases as 'Jewish' will 'fan the flames of popular anti-Semitism'.

A second criticism of knowledge arising from genetic research is that it could lead to Jews being labelled as more ill and prone to disease than other groups (Foster and Sharp 2002, Gilman 2006). The Jewish body has often been the 'case study for racial or genetic difference' and associating Jews with illness was another way in which Jews were differentiated from their Christian neighbours and reified as different (Gilman 2003: x). According to Gilman (2003), current genetic research into Ashkenazi Jews has led to the reappearance of nineteenth-century notions of an 'ill' Jewish body; the only difference is that illness is now seen to be the consequence of genetically transmitted diseases. Labelling diseases as 'Jewish' creates the impression that mainly Jews carry these diseases, and the reality is that a collective cannot carry a disease, only individuals can (Gilman 2003). Population and medical geneticists would be the first to point out that population genetics is about the overall average incidence of disease across different groups and does not mean that every individual within that group is at increased risk. However, this can easily be misinterpreted by members of the public, who may come to view all those belonging to a group as being at increased risk, as will become evident in this chapter. Gilman reminds us that diabetes was once considered to be a disease of the Jews and Africans, and this has now been shown to be incorrect. According to him:

> In the long run, it is probably better if Jews are spared the label of being an 'ill people', and for all individuals, Jewish or not, to undergo genetic testing

to at least identify those potential illnesses that they or their children may have, independent of their self-definition as 'Jews'.

(Gilman 2006: 2)

Concerns were raised, following the discovery of the Ashkenazi BRCA founder mutations in the mid-1990s, about the risks for Jews of being involved with genetic research. A 1999 resolution passed by the United Synagogue, representing Conservative Judaism in the United States, stated:

The Jewish community recognizes the interest of both the scientific and biotechnology community in expanding their knowledge base in the quest to understand, prevent and cure genetic diseases and, at the same time, the Jewish community has a strong interest in abating fear and avoiding stigmatization or discrimination.

(United Synagogue of Conservative Judaism 1999)

It is not my intention to discount these criticisms as they are important, often may be justified, and we should be cautious of current genetic research. However, most concerns are based almost exclusively on historical misuses of genetics and I want to examine this issue from a different angle. First, I use empirical data with high-risk women (and some non-high-risk men) to explore how they actually feel about/interpret contemporary research and clinical practices rather than relying on historical misuses. It is essential to point out that the data presented relates to how the Ashkenazi men and women interviewed personally felt towards genetic knowledge pertaining to Jews. Importantly, this does not address the possibility of discrimination by those outside the group (a topic that does arise) and, as we will see, there is evidence that there may be unintended consequences for how Jews are viewed both from within and by those outside the group. What this chapter reveals, however, is that these unintended or potentially harmful consequences are not necessarily experienced as problematic by the very individuals who are deemed to be high risk or belong to high-risk populations.

Continuities with historical discrimination

When a woman is first referred to a genetics clinic, it is standard clinical practice to send her a family history questionnaire. This questionnaire investigates the types and ages of cancer diagnoses in the family and is used to assess a woman's individual risk level. All questionnaires contain a question about whether you are Ashkenazi Jewish; this is consistent with the National Institute for Health and Clinical Excellence (NICE 2005) guidelines, which list Ashkenazi Jewish ancestry as an important risk factor. Elizabeth was a young unmarried woman in her early thirties who was born in Ukraine and had lived in Germany and Israel before moving to the UK. Elizabeth's mother and younger sister had breast cancer, and Elizabeth underwent BRCA testing but no mutation was found. Elizabeth was initially apprehensive when the family history questionnaire enquired about her Ashkenazi background:

> I had all different thoughts, thinking why would they ask me that? And how did they guess? [laughter] Like wow world conspiracy against us, what's going on? … 'Cuz the first idea is like every or many Jews who are paranoic [*sic*] pretty much about oh my God, 1929 [*sic*] has come back, oh my God, they are asking me now if I am Jewish and looking at my illnesses and they're gonna stereotype … but that didn't seem logical to me … but I had weird stuff going through my head but I didn't really feel discomfort or anything like that because … thinking about it longer obviously you do change your mind and it's not really possible that NHS [National Health Service] would be after that really. You know if I really did feel uncomfortable completely I probably wouldn't have answered it.

For Elizabeth, being asked if she was Ashkenazi Jewish on the family history questionnaire was reminiscent of the Second World War, Germany and historical discrimination. Despite her initial apprehension, she does not believe that there is a more sinister reason for requesting this information and in fact feels particularly protected because it is being asked by the NHS and relates to medical information. She distinguishes the abuses of the past from current medicine and research practices in which she places more trust.

Laura was a divorced British lawyer in her early fifties with no children who had been successfully treated and undergone a double mastectomy for breast cancer. She had been tested and no BRCA mutation was found. Laura said:

> I don't know if there's been any additional racism because African Caribbeans have sickle cell anemia or Greeks have thalassemia or Jews have Tay-Sachs. I think it's a no go area for most people. Children with disabilities is a no go area, don't think even the worst racists go that far. Well of course the worst racists, the Nazis did. Bad enough you're a Jew but they were also against disabled people. But I don't think … there is any overt racism about it but then that's only my view. But I've never come across it.

Laura acknowledges the past but does not actually feel at risk of such discrimination currently. The fact that most current genetic research focuses on diseases contributes to the view that it is beneficial because it offers the possibility of preventing disease and improving health. Anna was a British woman in her mid-forties with a strong family history of breast cancer. She was awaiting the results of her genetic test and also thought the benefits of knowing outweighed any potential negative consequences. For her, the personalized nature of the information made it particularly relevant:

> This is actually information that is about me. It's not about 20 per cent of the population, this is about me and I think that's great … I think that's a

unique opportunity, you know not many people get that opportunity. So it's not that I'm ashamed, you know I wouldn't see that at all, I think the only type of people that I would talk about it to certainly wouldn't be thinking 'oh Jewish background'. I certainly hope I wouldn't know anybody that would be thinking like that, that's for sure! [laughter] … so I think that would be the ill educated, or … the bigoted, yeah, you know there's always gonna be plenty of those around.

While Anna acknowledges that it is possible for some people, such as the 'ill educated' or 'bigoted', to make negative associations between being Jewish and having disease, she does not feel personally at risk of such discrimination and values the information giving her personal, and specific, data about her.

For most individuals, the topic of genetic research inevitably brought up the Jewish history of discrimination, persecution and the Holocaust. Importantly, while individuals were clearly aware of and sensitive to the historical misuses of genetics, they were not concerned about current genetics representing a continuation or renewal of the way in which scientific research or biological thinking had been used in the past. In fact, health-related research appeared to be conceptually separated, and therefore relatively protected, from these concerns. Overall, individuals felt the benefits of disease research outweighed any concerns regarding renewed discrimination.

Daniel was an unmarried successful retired businessman in his late forties whom I met while attending a lecture series at the London Jewish Cultural Centre. He did not have a family history of disease and our interview focused on Jewish identity and genetics in general. He was familiar with Tay-Sachs and told me that if he decided to marry, he would go for testing with his potential wife. He believed genetic research was very important:

> I think it would be ludicrous not to do this work … I mean scientific discovery … if one can do it without causing obvious pain and so on, why would we not explore beyond what is the genome made of? Why wouldn't we then apply that knowledge? Why would we not try and find cures for diseases if we can? Or for that matter understand growth and ageing? Why would we not? It's insane not to. And if there were useful categorizations that come … I don't understand why we would want to shut down those areas of knowledge … And if it can be tied to categories and groups, or diet, or culture, well okay culture is a step away from science, but if you can be clear about your knowledge and the causation then it's up to you what you make of it.

Daniel strongly supports scientific discovery, especially in relation to disease, even if it pertains to specific groups of people. Like Anna and Laura, Daniel distinguishes between research that is health or disease related and research that is not. He did comment that research into 'psychology or behaviour' might potentially be a cause for more concern or more difficult to justify, but he felt supportive and protective of health-related research.

All the individuals and organizations that I encountered during my research were extremely supportive and felt it was important to know as much as possible about disease among Ashkenazi Jews. This even extended to my own research; all of the individuals interviewed had a positive attitude and expressed gratitude that this research was being carried out. For example, at the end of my interview with Lori, she said: 'I'm really glad that you're doing research on it.'

Associating Ashkenazi Jews with ill health

This section turns to the second main concern regarding genetic research into Ashkenazi Jews, that they will be considered or labelled as more ill or prone to disease. In this case, a more nuanced picture emerges as there was evidence that women did interpret genetic breast cancer as a Jewish woman's disease and had an exaggerated sense of risk for all Jewish women, which could be reinforced through clinical encounters. Sarah was a well-known American author in her late forties who had lived in London for over 20 years. She had been successfully treated for breast cancer two years earlier. She had three sisters, two of whom also had breast cancer; one of her sisters had survived but the other had unfortunately died. Sarah's third sister was taking Tamoxifen prophylactically (a hormonal drug treatment that can be prescribed to help prevent breast cancer for some high-risk women). Sarah, her mother and one surviving sister had all been tested for BRCA mutations but none had been identified in the family. Sarah's geneticist had told her that her family was 'clearly a BRCA2 family' but they just could not find the mutation in Sarah's case, leaving her certain that the breast cancers in her family were genetic. This belief was reinforced by her geneticist, who mentioned the possibility of a BRCA3 gene that had not yet been discovered. Sarah's clinical encounters led her to reinterpret her risk in relation to being Ashkenazi Jewish:

> I always sort of thought of it as my family. I didn't so much recognize it as a *cultural affliction* ... I mean I knew when I started going for mammograms, people did ask, always asked on the questionnaires that you filled in before – 'are you from an Ashkenazi Jewish family?' So then you start to become aware that this is, this is a thing, something people are noticing. [emphasis added]

For some women, such as Elizabeth, a clinical appointment or filling out the family history questionnaire was the first time they became aware that perhaps there was a connection between their risk and being Ashkenazi:

> When I arrived at the clinic, usually in this country they would ask you for your ethnic background and we usually say White, and one of the

questions was … are you Ashkenazi Jew? And … I stopped for a moment and I thought why don't they ask whether I'm Asian Bengali or something? Why are they asking me? This is strange. So I did have to put a cross on yes. I returned the questionnaire and actually spoke to my mom on that day, saying 'you know what's strange? They're asking you, this is weird'.

Rachel was an American-born woman in her late forties whose sister was a BRCA1 mutation carrier with breast cancer. She had not decided if she was going to undergo genetic testing. In the clinic, she found herself surrounded by staff who were aware of the risk and this left her feeling slightly singled out:

> I didn't know everybody else knew it. In the sense, not the genetic counsellor as much as the women who did the mammogram knew it and that's what seemed strange. I felt like loads of people know this and I never really knew it and I am Jewish and they're not Jewish and it's like well how come they know it? … But it feels like being labelled. … only 'cuz suddenly I'm fitting into some category and I'm not used to being slotted into.

Rachel describes feeling slightly 'singled out' during her clinical encounters, and surprised by how many clinical staff knew of the risks for Ashkenazi Jews (further discussion of Rachel's story can be found in chapters four and five). Other women described experiences where doctors had told them or friends that Ashkenazi Jews were more sick or prone to disease. Sarah recounted a story where she had gone to a dinner party and been talking to a doctor who was interested in genetics. When he found out she was Ashkenazi Jewish, he told her that Ashkenazi Jews had a higher incidence of breast cancer and depression, and also had a 'music gene' and a gene for increased intelligence. Sarah believed that Jews had these afflictions, and abilities, in higher incidence: 'Intelligence, music, breast cancer, depression. Two good, two bad, I'm sure there are lots of others.'

Perhaps this doctor was familiar with recent studies that suggest the conglomeration of genetic diseases at increased incidence among Ashkenazi Jews have remained at a high frequency because they provide a beneficial effect of increased intelligence (Cochran et al. 2005, Murray 2007). This genetic theory proposes that because Jews were historically banned from owning land and Christianity forbade usury, many Jews ended up being moneylenders. These jobs required intelligence and mathematical literacy, and the recessive diseases that occur with increased frequency among Ashkenazi Jews all involve the neuronal systems of the brain. This is another example of how genetic explanations for disease reiterate collective Ashkenazi history. The population geneticist David Goldstein (2008: 110) refers to these studies as 'tantalizing, circumstantial, politically incorrect in the extreme, and entirely speculative'; yet he concludes the argument cannot be ruled out and requires formal testing.

Michelle was a religiously observant British woman in her late thirties. She was married with two children and worked part time from home. Her mother had breast cancer five years earlier, and she had attended a genetic clinic for advice about genetic testing but not yet undergone testing. She told me that when her mother visited her doctor for a regular breast check up, her doctor sent her for a mammogram because Ashkenazi Jewish women have the highest percentage of breast cancer. Ashkenazi Jewish women have the highest incidence of genetic breast cancer, but this is not the same as having the highest percentage of breast cancer, as this doctor implied. Nancy, a married British woman in her early forties with a family history of breast cancer, recounted a story about her Ashkenazi Jewish friend who went to see her doctor for colitis. Her doctor reportedly said: 'What do you expect? You're Ashkenazi Jewish.' Women were getting messages from doctors, clinical encounters and family history questionnaires that Ashkenazi Jews were more prone to illness than others, which reinforced the idea that all Ashkenazi women were at risk. Anna's younger sister, Susan, was also awaiting the result of her BRCA mutation test. According to Susan: 'Every time another person gets it in our community it's just, you know, the way it's going to be.'

Susan's view illustrates how an increased risk for a population can easily become confused with an increased risk for all individuals within that population, a belief that Laura also expressed. Laura's breast cancer was unusual in that it was not related to her family history but to treatment she had undergone as a teenager for Hodgkin's disease. The heavy doses of radiation to her chest that were commonly used during the 1960s had severely increased her risk of developing breast cancer. Laura did also have a family history of cancer, with her grandmother and great aunt having the disease, but it was not thought to be related to her own breast cancer. Despite this, Laura had undergone testing for the Ashkenazi mutations in the BRCA genes on the advice of her geneticist:

> So the chances of me having the BRCA1 and BRCA2 were quite remote. Well I could've had them as an Ashkenazi woman, but we knew that wasn't the cause but I was tested anyways because Dr M was very keen … and my oncologist … she knew that Dr M was interested in Ashkenazi women.

Her story demonstrates the willingness of geneticists to test Ashkenazi women even when the family history is not particularly strong. The fact that Laura's clinician suggested she be tested despite her cancer not being related to her family history may have contributed to her belief that all Ashkenazi Jewish women were at risk:

> It looks like breast cancer is an epidemic … and the general population have a 1 in 10 chance of getting it … But for Jewish women, Ashkenazi women it's worse! It's a dead cert. Look at your neighbour either side and they're gonna get it.

Laura was surprised that they had been unable to find a mutation in her family:

> We don't have the BRCA and we're Ashkenazi, pure Ashkenazi women as well ... And that's a huge sample of Ashkenazi men and women from one family so you'd think you'd be able to tell a lot ... it's very surprising there aren't any BRCA genes.

Laura believes that simply because she is Ashkenazi it is likely that a mutation would be found in her family. The population risk is misunderstood as individual risk. These beliefs (whether accurate or not) about heightened risk did not present a problem for the women interviewed and instead provided an opportunity to use this knowledge to empower women, increase awareness and prevent breast cancer in future. Laura described a sense of duty she felt when attending her local gym to undress in front of other women and not be embarrassed about her mastectomy. She felt this was a way of increasing awareness and helping to inform other Jewish women. She even tried to organize an information session at her local gym but the manager was not particularly interested. Laura was so keen to raise awareness that she suggested we write an article together for the *Jewish Chronicle* newspaper. Women took ownership of the increased risk and believed it was something that all Ashkenazi women needed to know about, and some women, such as Michelle, suggested population screening without knowing about the current projects that were under way (described in chapter two).

> To me the better knowledge you have, the better you can deal with the situation ... so I think ... if you knew that that gene was the *risky gene* as an Ashkenazi woman, I think if you could have it tested privately, I don't need to because Hospital X will do it, but if you could go privately I'd have it done, definitely. [emphasis added]

Even if Michelle were not eligible for testing under the National Health Service, which she is, she would have it done privately and suggests this is something that all Ashkenazi women should do. Michelle believed all Ashkenazi women should be tested and recommended adding it to Tay-Sachs screening programmes:

> And again if someone said to me, oh whilst you're having your test for Tay-Sachs, would you like me to test you? Well okay, while you're taking the blood, test it for whatever you like. It's just the knowledge isn't it? It's like with anything if you're forewarned, you're forearmed.

Michelle's familiarity with Tay-Sachs screening, which she underwent before marriage, made it easy for her to imagine just adding the test on to this pre-existing programme, despite the significant differences between the diseases in terms of transmission, severity, lethality, age of onset and the treatments available. Sarah expressed a similar view:

> I mean information, information is important. What you do with it is the question then, isn't it? But I don't think ignorance is at all good. I mean all this talk about breast cancer screening, you know why not screen the populations that are at higher risk?

Jennifer was the first cousin of Anna and Susan. She was in her early forties and was awaiting her genetics appointment. Jennifer was another woman who, like Laura, thought it was crucial to let all Jewish women know about their risk and that 'rabbis in their pulpits should be telling women'. She did not see this as something that would cause alarm or make women worried but rather that it left women 'empowered' and 'in control'. When I asked Jennifer if she had any concerns about research being specifically focused on Ashkenazi Jews, she replied:

> Oh no, I'm in favour of that. I am totally in favour of it. If it can help in any way to shed light ... why not? I think it's a good thing, I don't mind that at all. No it doesn't bother me in the least ... I think all Ashkenazi Jewish women should know because then they can really you know do something positive. I mean I see this as a very positive thing ... I don't see it as alarming people, I just see it as informing people and then once you're informed it's up to you to make your choice.

The doctor whom Jennifer saw at her local hospital had warned her that she might have to face some 'awful decisions' and that genetic testing could be a 'double-edged sword' because she might have to consider a prophylactic mastectomy if she was found to be a carrier. Her clinician's ambivalence about the value of the test did not deter Jennifer at all. She believed that it was better to know, although she acknowledged that her mother and some of her cousins did not feel the same way and preferred not to undergo genetic testing.

The following section presents the survey data and what knowledge a non-high-risk sample of Ashkenazi Jews had about the BRCA mutations. Again, a generally positive and supportive attitude towards research and testing was reflected by the survey respondents.

BRCA survey results

Over 200 surveys were distributed and the response rate was over 50 per cent (111 surveys returned). The mean age of survey respondents was 60, with the youngest respondent being 20 and the oldest being 80 years of age. Almost all respondents (93 per cent) were female. Of the total sample, 77 per cent were over 50 and the remaining 23 per cent under 50. Three-quarters of respondents were married (74 per cent) and 81 per cent had children. Respondents had a high educational level, with half the respondents having undergraduate or postgraduate degrees (20 per cent and 30 per cent respectively). Nearly half (40 per cent) were in paid employment. One drawback of the survey is that it did not directly ask about concerns with being the subjects of genetic research, such as those related to discrimination. This was not deemed suitable or ethical given the self-completed nature of the survey and the fact that awareness levels regarding genetic disease or research were completely unknown. However, respondents were given space for any additional comments they wanted to make at the end of the survey. The only comments left by respondents expressed support for my own research, to indicate how important this research was, and the need to continue research in general and raise awareness of the genetic breast cancer risk among Ashkenazi Jews. Survey respondents were keen to help with my research and over half (54 per cent) agreed to be contacted in future for an interview. This supports the qualitative interview data where individuals expressed an overridingly supportive attitude towards research focused on Ashkenazi Jews.

Survey respondents had high awareness levels of the BRCA genes: nearly two-thirds of women (63 per cent) had heard of the BRCA genes, while the remaining 37 per cent had heard 'nothing' about them. The highest proportion of individuals who had knowledge of the genes had received it from the media (41 per cent). Nearly one-quarter had sought advice from a doctor regarding genetic testing, the majority for Tay-Sachs or cancer. Of the total number of respondents, 10 per cent had been diagnosed with breast cancer, which is consistent with the general breast cancer incidence of approximately one in nine women (Cancer Research UK 2008). Three women had undergone BRCA mutation testing, representing 3 per cent of the total sample. All of the women tested had personal or family histories of breast cancer and ranged in age from 50 to 67, with two of the women being 50 years old. Of the three women tested, two were found not to be carriers and one had an inconclusive result.

The survey included a series of eight true/false/not sure questions intended to measure knowledge about the genes, which was based on Lerman et al.'s (1996) 11-item scale to assess understanding about BRCA mutation testing. The final question asked if Ashkenazi Jews were at increased risk of carrying mutations in the genes. Over half of respondents were aware of the increased risk (53 per cent), while 42 per cent were not sure; only a very small number believed that Ashkenazi Jews were not at increased risk (3 per cent). It is difficult to interpret responses to true/false/not sure questions, as individuals had already been asked about genetic testing and family history of cancer so they may have deduced that there was an increased risk for Ashkenazi Jews and responded true because of these previous questions. However, the responses indicate a fairly high awareness level of the increased risk for Ashkenazi Jews, which is consistent with the high number of women who reported having knowledge of the genes (63 per cent).

Conclusion

Critics of contemporary genetics often use the historical exploitations and abuses of genetics as warnings of the risks of pursuing such research currently (Braun et al. 2007, Caulfield et al. 2009, Gilman 2006, Obasogie 2009). When the historical context is taken into account, it is easy to understand why social science commentary is often highly critical or deeply suspicious (Rose 2007: 39) of developments regarding population/race, genetics and illness. One of the major criticisms of genetic medicine and testing focused on Ashkenazi Jews is that it will lead to a re-emergence of historical forms of discrimination and anti-Semitism (Gilman 1985, 2003, Glenn 2010). As a researcher, I also had a personal expectation that I would find some disquiet among women about discrimination or stigmatization.

While it is important not to neglect the past, this chapter has attempted to approach the subject from a different standpoint. First, it has explored this issue from the perspective of high-risk women. By focusing on empirical data, the chapter has directed our attention to the experiences of individual members of high-risk populations, and simultaneously avoided the temptation to use the 'lessons of history' as the sole basis for critiques of population genetic research. On one level, the qualitative data presented here does not support such concerns and highlights that individual experience may differ significantly from concerns which are based solely on the historical record. While the Jewish history of discrimination and Nazi persecution arose in most interviews and individuals were sensitive to this past, current genetic research and medicine were not viewed as a continuation of historical discrimination. In contrast, women were not particularly concerned about being discriminated against or being labelled as ill. Instead, they were supportive of genetic medicine and testing and believed it was a valuable pursuit that provided useful information that could help ensure the health of Jews. It did not make women less supportive of research or create fears about being categorized as sick, but had the opposite effect. This supports Cowan's (2008) suggestion that we must separate contemporary genetic testing from the 'old eugenics' of the twentieth century. Contemporary medical genetics is a pronatalist endeavour intended to reduce suffering, motivated from below by the people most affected by it rather than mandated from above by governments, as eugenic programmes were (Cowan 2008). Those interviewed clearly separated current medical genetics from prior abuses, and concerns about continuities with historical discrimination or Nazi eugenics were not reflected in individual accounts.

However, and importantly, there was evidence that clinical encounters and family history questionnaires have the potential to leave women with an exaggerated sense that all Ashkenazi Jewish women are at risk of genetic breast cancer and more prone to disease than other groups of people. While this belief may not have been a problem for the women themselves, it does indicate that entire groups can become linked with disease and there may be a possibility of discrimination or stigmatization by non-Jews. Not only lay individuals but also medical professionals can easily misunderstand the differences between population risk and individual risk. One consequence of Ashkenazi Jews' historical support for and participation in genetic research and screening programmes is that they have become over-represented in genetic research findings, with research continually building upon the pre-existing body of literature and samples. In this context, diseases easily become 'Jewish diseases' even though little may be known about mutation frequencies in other populations (Azoulay 2003, Birenbaum Carmeli 2004, Wailoo and Pemberton 2006). When individual disease genes, such as the 'Ashkenazi BRCA mutations', are designated as Jewish because they are statistically more common in Jews, this can lead to an 'easy conceptual slippage' (Kahn 2005: 13) whereby all individuals are mistakenly associated with that disease. Although not necessarily problematic for Jewish women, one consequence is that genetic breast cancer can itself become a 'Jewish disease', and this raises questions about how others might interpret knowledge about disease among Ashkenazi Jews.

The over-representation of Ashkenazi Jews should also alert us to the question of representation in general and the uneven ways in which genetic medicine may be developing in relation to population. Populations such as Ashkenazi Jews, whose over-representation has led to a great deal of knowledge and information about them, may derive additional benefits from new developments, drug targets and the high level of knowledge about their specific diseases or genetic predispositions. In contrast, those populations who are under-represented may lose out due to the lack of knowledge about them. In the US, African Americans and Hispanics are insufficiently represented in BRCA clinical services and testing (as well as many other health care arenas). This under-representation has worsened health disparities, and researchers are concerned that the lack of data for particular populations may make the available data less relevant (Mozersky and Joseph 2010). Of course, this assumes that genetic knowledge will provide important treatment and prevention options. However, increasing efforts to develop personalized medicine (that is, medicine based on individual or population genetic profiling) could mean that those who are not represented in research will not stand to gain from the potential benefits that may arise.

While genetic research undoubtedly comes with gifts and poisons (Taussig et al. 2003), we should be cautious before labelling entire groups or populations as vulnerable to the consequences of medical research. Luna's (2009) concept of 'layers of vulnerability' is a useful analytical and conceptual tool here. Luna (2009: 122) is concerned with the conception of 'vulnerable groups' in research ethics and the tendency to use vulnerability as a 'fixed label on a particular subpopulation'. She critiques the homogenizing and stereotyping effects of labelling an entire population as 'vulnerable', and proposes conceiving of vulnerability as layered, dynamic and situational. While it is crucial not to neglect the fact that there may indeed be vulnerable individuals within a group, or that a person can be rendered vulnerable depending on their circumstances, it is just as important to remember that no population is essentially vulnerable. Even for a group such as Ashkenazi Jews, with a long history of discrimination and stigmatization at times based on a supposed propensity for disease and ill health, genetic medicine is not necessarily interpreted in predictable ways.

The following chapter moves beyond discrimination to explore the impact that knowledge of an elevated genetic risk had on women's Jewish self-identity. Specifically this chapter examines the ways in which Jewish identity is conceptualized and the importance of biological concepts in forging Jewish identity, and how this conception plays an important role in the way in which genetic information is interpreted and received by Ashkenazi Jews.

4 On being Jewish

Despite the fact that bioethicists have sounded every conceivable caution about the social and political dangers of conceptualizing Jewishness in genetically essentialized terms, and despite the fact that anthropologists have argued for decades that identity is socially constructed, contemporary Jews seem to be finding the concept of the Jewish gene irresistible.

(Kahn 2005: 14)

The previous chapters demonstrated that there are unintended consequences – both beneficial and potentially harmful – to being involved in genetic research. Despite warnings that genetic research into Ashkenazi Jews could lead to discrimination or Jews being labelled as ill (Azoulay 2003, Donelle et al. 2005, Foster and Sharp 2002, Gilman 2003, 2006, Kahn 2005), individuals were not concerned about these things but rather saw genetics as a way to help ensure the health of Ashkenazi Jews. However, I want to go further in examining this apparently supportive attitude, and in this chapter I explore Jewish identity and the multiple ways in which belonging is conceptualized. The chapter builds upon and offers new insight into the large body of literature that argues genetic technologies, and the ability to predict who is at risk of future disease, will have a significant impact on the way in which individuals see themselves or the groups to which they belong (Brodwin 2002, Finkler 2001, Hallowell 1999, Novas and Rose 2000, Rabinow 1996, Rapp 2000). For Novas and Rose (2000: 485) genetics and genetic medicine are leading to a 'mutation in personhood' that affects how individuals conceive of themselves and their bodies. When an individual goes for a genetic consultation, this involves a 'genetic re-mapping where the individual reconfigures their identity in terms of a genetic past, a genetic present and a genetic future', and individuals may come to see themselves in a genetic way (Novas and Rose 2000: 495). Novas and Rose qualify their claims by stating that genetic identity is operating within a much larger and highly complex field of identity practices that include identity claims such as nationality, culture, sexuality, religion, dietary choice and many others. Rather than supplanting these multiple and plural identity claims, biological and genetic identity will 'infuse, interact [with], combine [with] and contest' (Novas and Rose 2000: 491) these other identities.

Finkler (2000) is particularly interested in how contemporary genetic disease inheritance orients people to kinship and family. According to Finkler (2000), contemporary Western society is marked by an ideology of choice and it is those with whom we choose to share our household and love that define our family and kin relations. However, knowledge of genetic disease has led to a resurgence of the biological importance of kin and family and is effecting a return to notions of kinship based on consanguinity rather than choice. Family and kin relationships are being drawn into the biomedical domain through our current understanding that disease genes are transmitted from generation to generation, what Finkler calls the medicalization of kinship (Finkler 2000: 3). Finkler (2001: 237) acknowledges that kinship and family ties based on blood are usually a 'mark of specific ethnicity and traditionalism' and may still be very strong for some ethnic groups, yet she goes no further in addressing the relationship between medical genetics and ethnic groups, something this research is particularly concerned with.

Much of the discussion about the impact of genetic research and knowledge on Jewish identity has suggested that it will lead to a privileging of biological identity over other social mechanisms that lead to collective identity, and that referring to 'Jewish' genes and diseases naturalizes Jews as a biological group when in reality they are actually a social group (Azoulay 2003, Brodwin 2002, Kahn 2005, Neulander 2006). The material presented in this chapter contributes to and extends the above claims regarding genetics and identity. In particular, women's and men's narratives about Jewish identity reveal a complex and nuanced picture, one where biological and social concepts are so interwoven that they are virtually inseparable. The concept of co-production (Jasanoff 2004) remains a useful tool especially because by giving primacy to neither the natural nor the social it is possible to see how the two are mutually con- stituted. At the same time, I want to probe further about what exactly the 'biolo- gical' means when we speak of 'biological' identity. When the 'biological' parts of identity are social themselves, or at least inseparable and co-produced alongside the 'social', these very categories and distinctions are called into question.

Interview material from non-high-risk individuals, including men, is included in this chapter as it helps to illustrate the multifaceted ways in which Jewish belonging is conceptualized, even for those without genetic disease.

Jewish conceptions of kinship and belonging

The question of who is a Jew and what constitutes 'Jewishness' is one of the most vexed and contested issues of modern religious and ethnic group history (Glenn and Sokoloff 2010). The two traditional routes to Judaism are matri- lineal descent or conversion. According to Jewish law, it is necessary to have a Jewish mother in order to be considered Jewish, although more liberal branches of Judaism no longer necessarily adhere to this. There is a long history of debate within Judaism regarding the basis of Jewishness itself (Kahn 2000). On the one hand, Jewish philosophers have argued Jewishness is the result of divine election, physiological differences or kinship, while others have argued Jewishness is nothing more than the product of commitment to and observance of the Jewish religion. Judaism has never been a proselytizing religion; while conversion is possible, it is a difficult process and is meant to be so in order to ensure the convert is committed (Kahn 2000). Conversion does not account for a large proportion of those who consider themselves Jews but there are indeed converts to Judaism. The fact that Judaism accepts converts is often cited as evidence that Judaism cannot be biological (Kahn 2000: 1–2). At the same time, traditional Jewish law requires that one has a Jewish mother in order to be considered Jewish. As Kahn (2000) points out, this results in an ever present conceptual tension wherein Judaism appears to be both the product of kinship and the product of commitment. The importance of having a Jewish mother for establishing someone as Jewish should not be understated, and this is often one of the differentiating features between the various religious movements within Judaism. The UK Orthodox movement does not recognize children of non-Jewish mothers as being Jewish, whereas Liberal and Reform synagogues have more inclusive views regarding who can be considered Jewish, including those with patrilineal lineage. Until the mid-twentieth century, Jews tended to marry other Jews and often lived together in Jewish communities, so the question of who was a Jew was not a particularly significant one (Markel 1997). Increasing rates of intermarriage and the rising number of Jews not traditionally considered Jewish, such as those with Jewish fathers but not mothers, have made the issue more salient today and exacerbated the difficulty of defining who is a Jew.

This question of who is considered a Jew became headline news around the world in a case that was brought to Britain's Supreme Court in 2009 (Lyall 2009, Weiler 2010). The legal case was initiated by the parents of a child who was denied admission to a large Jewish secondary school in London. The child and his parents were religiously observant Jews, but the boy's mother had converted to Judaism. The conversion had not taken place within the Orthodox United Synagogue but through the more liberal UK Jewish movement known as Masorti. Non-Orthodox conversions are not officially recognized by the United Synagogue. The school, which has a long waiting list, denied the boy entry as he was not considered Jewish. The United Synagogue's chief representative, Lord Rabbi Jonathan Sacks, supported the school's decision based on the fact that 'membership' of the Jewish people rather than 'practice' defined who was Jewish. The family sued the school and the case eventually made its way up to the Supreme Court, where it was ruled that the requirement of having a Jewish mother in order to be considered Jewish was in fact racial discrimination. The court distinguished between religious and racial/ethnic discrimination. In the UK, it is legal to deny entry to a religious organization on the basis of religion, and therefore Jewish students can be offered places ahead of non-Jewish students when there is oversubscription. However, denying entry or admission based on 'race or ethnicity' is illegal; the court ruled that religion was a result of practice/observance, while being born to a Jewish mother was 'ethnic' and therefore it was illegal for the school to deny the boy entrance based on this requirement. This case, among other things, highlights the ongoing tensions and difficulties in defining who is a Jew and the overlapping and unclear boundaries of race, ethnicity and 'biological' and 'social' forms of identity. It also illustrates how biology and culture are dichotomized as clearly separable domains, with biology being explicitly linked to birth and blood (and therefore race or ethnicity) while practice or observance is considered 'cultural' or 'social' (and therefore religion).

The notion that Jews are a biological group has been more or less emphasized at different historical times and been a reflection of the broader social context or political aims. It is important to recognize the ways in which the scientific endeavour may be influenced by the social and ideological context in which it occurs (Jasanoff 2004, Kirsh 2003). From the mid-nineteenth to the early twentieth century, biological concepts of race and ethnicity were ubiquitous and held by most people, including physicians, social reformers, civil servants, academics and businessmen. During this period, many Jews and Jewish scientists held the view that Jews were a biologically separate group and were comfortable with arguments, claims and research into the heritable traits and racial difference of the Jews (Endelman 2004). Jewish scientists and Jews in general were supportive of eugenics at this time, in the sense of encouraging the 'fittest' or healthiest to reproduce and so ensure a strong future population and discouraging those who were not from reproducing (Endelman 2004: 67). Eugenic notions fit with the pre-existing eugenic framework present in Judaism that encourages the careful selection of marriage partners, often through matchmaking, and a high reproductive rate (Endelman 2004). During this period, discussions, research, lectures and articles proliferated on the Jewish race, Jewish traits and Jewish heritability. One prominent Jewish British scientist named Redcliffe Salaman (1874–1955) was particularly interested in Jewish genetics, and his research even extended to the ability to recognize Jews by their facial characteristics. British Jews of the time believed that both religion and race were central to defining Jewishness. This was a period when religious practice and devotion were declining because assimilation and intermarriage were increasing and so biological claims about the nature of Jewishness were useful to support the notion that being Jewish was a result of more than just ritual observance (Endelman 2004).

Not all British Jewish scientists were comfortable with claims about Jewish biological difference because of fears regarding the potential for discrimination, but until the early 1930s they did not form the majority. The rise of Nazism in the 1930s significantly altered this and most Jewish scientists rejected all notions of a biological basis to Jewishness in response to Nazi ideology. A report by the Jewish Health Organisation of Great Britain in 1934 claimed that there was 'no such thing as a Jewish race in the biological use of the word' (Endelman 2004: 80) despite the fact that it had previously endorsed biological research into Jews. Following the Holocaust, the idea that race was merely a social construct with no biological basis dominated most discourse for many years (as described in the introduction).

In Israel, however, the ideological and social context influenced the scientific endeavour very differently (Kirsh 2003). Kirsh (2003) has shown that post-Second World War Israeli geneticists and physicians were influenced by Zionist ideology that penetrated their scientific activity. Israeli scientists at this time stressed certain aspects of their work, and presented their results, so as to confirm the common historical and biological origins of Jews and maintain religious, genetic and national Jewish identity. For instance, scientists minimized results that suggested differences between 'communities' of Jews, and emphasized the common origins of Jews. There was an avoidance of speculation about intermarriage and maintenance of the idea that consanguineous marriage led to a high frequency of certain genes, with terms such as 'gene influx' being used instead of intermarriage. This had the result of leaving the Jewish gene pool 'pure and unalterable' (Kirsh 2003: 648). According to Kirsh (2003), Israeli scientists' explanations were biased by their adherence to a pre-existing narrative and did not take into account other possible, and equally plausible, interpretations of their data. The language used in scientific articles included referring to Jews as brothers or tribes and using biblical references that implied and assumed a common biological origin and 'non interrupted genealogical ties' among Jews (Kirsh 2003: 650). While not denying that Israeli scientists and geneticists in the period between 1950 and 1963 were serious and conscientious scientists whose work was peer reviewed, appeared in international medical journals and was cited by others, Kirsh (2003: 655) argues that Israeli scientists were guided by an 'invisible hand' that was the 'internalized image of their history and nationality'. According to Hashiloni-Dolev (2006: 142), Zionism can itself be thought of as a 'eugenicist project' that argued there was a biological essence or aspect to Jewishness. This view was contested, in the wake of the Holocaust, by other European Jews fighting racism and the idea that Jews were a race. Thus for Israeli society 'the problematic history of medical genetics, with its fatal consequences for the European Jews, had gone entirely unnoticed' (Hashiloni-Dolev 2006: 142).

The notion that Jewishness is not biological retains great cultural force (Kahn 2005) and many people I encountered cited the Holocaust as the main reason why it was dangerous to refer to Jews as a race or in biological terms. Questions regarding the basis of Jewish belonging continue to this day and were common at the London Jewish Cultural Centre, where various events regarding Jewish identity were held, including lectures such as 'Judaism: An Exclusive Club?' and 'A Question of Identity'. At these events there would be a panel of speakers and the room was always full to capacity with a mixture of young and old. Issues discussed included the changing nature of Jewishness, the fact that many people no longer believe in God or ritually observe Judaism, the increase in intermarriage and the difficulties in using matrilineal descent to define who is Jewish. At one event a speaker very clearly stated that Judaism is not a race because humans are so similar genetically that this topic did not even warrant discussion. At another event some panel members said that Judaism must be a race because of the requirement to have a Jewish mother and therefore be 'born Jewish' regardless of whether one believes in the religion or not. Others disagreed strongly with this view, including one panel member who had only a Jewish father yet was religiously observant and considered himself to be completely Jewish.

The London Jewish Cultural Centre held a course devoted to the Cohen modal haplotype and mitochondrial DNA genetic studies (described in chapter two) called the 'Lost Jews of Africa'. The course was taught by the anthropologist Tudor Parfitt, who had been involved in some of the studies that had confirmed the Jewish identity of various groups in Asia and Africa (Thomas et al. 2000). Throughout the course there was a lot of discussion about whether Jews were a biological or cultural group, including an assignment to write about the role that biology played in our own Jewish identities. At the outset, the lecturer explained that race was meaningless as genetics had proven that there was more variation between two individuals than between any two groups. However, he explained, there are 'repeating patterns or markers found mostly in junk DNA' that tend to run in families or groups and can be used to reveal ethnic background. The lecturer acknowledged this apparent contradiction, the lack of boundaries in defining who is a Jew, and how using the word race could be problematic; yet at the same time the course was about the very ways in which genetics had been used to prove or disprove the Jewish identity of various groups.

In the following section I use the qualitative interview material to explore how individuals conceived of their own Jewish identity and the complex and contradictory role that biology played in defining Jewish belonging.

On being Jewish

I began most interviews by asking people to tell me about their Jewish upbringing and what role, if any, Judaism played in their lives currently. This would then usually open up a conversation regarding Jewish identity. It would generally emerge naturally over the course of the interview, rather than in response to a direct question, how people felt about being Jewish. I had initially thought that I could explicitly ask whether people thought being Jewish was cultural or biological, but this turned out to be an overly simplistic, and naive, plan. In one of my earliest interviews with Ben, a young British man in his mid-twenties with no family history of disease, I asked him directly about whether he thought of Jews as a biological or cultural group, to which he responded in a slightly confused manner: 'Um, are those the two options?' Ben did not see these as discrete and separate categories, and my question clearly imposed upon him a way of thinking about Jewishness that did not fit with his own experience:

> I would say even though it's the easy way out, a bit of both … if you just have some *Jewish blood* that basically means you're a Hebrew, because

for all intents and purposes it's part of your family lineage and that just makes sense to me, it's just common sense ... *I was born Jewish* and for better or worse that's just how it is ... it also seems to me that it's cultural ... it does seem to me that culture is the life experience, the rest is just the starting point. [emphasis added]

Ben felt uncomfortable describing Jews as a biological group because this could be interpreted as anti-Semitic or reminiscent of the Nazis: 'I suppose the connotation of the term biological just instinctively irks me and that's why maybe I have trouble using it.' Ben described his Jewishness as being a result of Jewish blood, lineage and birth, yet he was uncomfortable with the use of the words biology or race. At the same time, Ben felt that there was something 'distinctively Jewish' about many cultural and literary Jewish figures and the works they produced, and he wondered if this was related to the fact that they were 'born Jewish', because many of them were secular and assimilated Jews who did not ritually observe Judaism:

I wouldn't be able to define it in precise scientific terms ... it is something I feel many of those Jewish cultural figures had within them because they were born Jewish, and therefore had Jewish ancestry so that probably ties in with ... strictly speaking, the definition of what biological means.

For Ben, the qualities that Jewish cultural figures possessed were not a result of ritual observance, but rather something that was 'within them' and therefore the result of being 'born Jewish' or having Jewish ancestry. While Ben acknowledged that ancestry and birth might 'strictly speaking' be the definition of what biological means, he was not comfortable with this line of thinking. But if blood, lineage and birth are not biological, what are they? Or rather, what is biological? For Ben, being Jewish was a combination of being born Jewish, having Jewish blood, sharing ancestry as well as having certain cultural sensibilities and ways of understanding the world. These were neither cultural nor biological but an amalgamation of both and not conceptually separated. I stopped asking individuals this question in my later interviews.

Elana was a ritually observant British woman in her seventies who did not have a personal or family history of breast cancer. I was introduced to Elana by her grandson Michael, whom I also interviewed. Elana attended synagogue weekly and her late husband was a cantor, a trained musician and vocalist who leads the synagogue prayer services along with the rabbi. I spent the day with Elana at her home by the seaside and she described the nature of Jewishness to me: 'It is biological. It is. Obviously through the mother as you know.' Yet, at the same time, Elana explained to me that Judaism was the product of upbringing: 'While we remain distinct, we're a people ... We don't have children any differently to the non-Jewish people, it's how we bring them up and what we teach them from babyhood really.'

Elana explicitly uses the term biological to refer to the requirement of needing a Jewish mother and describes Jews as a 'people', yet she also simultaneously removes any biological difference by explaining that Judaism is a product of upbringing and not a result of having 'children any differently'. Elana's grandson Michael was a young religiously observant British student whom I met at the London Jewish Cultural Centre. During our interview he described the requirement of being 'born Jewish':

> I think it is difficult if you are not born into it ... Obviously culturally you can be Jewish and not technically be Jewish, but for me ... what is more important? Biologically because you can't get rid of that, culturally it is just a matter of choice ... if you're genetically Jewish and born genetically Jewish, you're never gonna lose that and ... you're stuck with it!

Michael's description presents a more explicitly dichotomized version of belonging, with being born Jewish as something genetic you cannot 'get rid of' and culture being a 'matter of choice':

> So I wouldn't say to be Jewish you have to um have a massive interest in Judaism or know anything because you can just be biologically Jewish ... but obviously I do come across people who haven't got a Jewish mother and they still think they are Jewish, and I say yeah that is fine okay in terms of religiously. I am probably not gonna marry you if you are a girl because *technically you are not really Jewish*. [emphasis added]

The idea that not being born to a Jewish mother meant that one was not 'technically' Jewish arose frequently. Daniel was another individual who told me about having friends who turned out to be 'Jews in some technical sense, meaning that it turns out that a stream of women in their family have all been Jewish'. He had one particular female friend who, despite being 'clearly Church of England', had been born to a Jewish mother but not raised as a Jew because her parents divorced when she was very young and she was raised by her Christian father. According to Daniel, this woman and her non-Jewish husband had 'blue eyed and stub nosed' children who were all 'technically Jewish'.

While people did not deny that those who converted or had only Jewish fathers could still be considered Jewish, there was a sense that somehow they were not really Jewish, at least not by blood and birth. Yet, in this conception, being Jewish requires being born to a Jewish mother and therefore having Jewish blood, but what happens to the other non-Jewish biological half (i.e. your father)? Put another way, if Jewish mothers lead to Jewish belonging, but Jewish fathers do not, then what is biology or Jewish blood?[1] It would not meet a biogenetic definition about genetic inheritance as a child inherits equal amounts of genetic material from both parents. So this is not a biological understanding of belonging that fits with biomedicine or science or genetics;

rather, it is a biological understanding that reiterates the social (see Kahn 2000). In describing the use of reproductive technologies in Israel, Kahn (2000: 169) refers to the 'cutting and pasting' of conceptual kinship and the ways in which biological facts can be 'erased' and social facts can be rearranged, especially when rabbis want to legitimate Jewish children conceived by unmarried Jewish women or infertile couples who use non-Jewish genetic material. Kahn accurately notes that any conjecture about the relationship between the social and the biological must be re-examined, because they are not coherent or stable.

Jennifer did not have a particularly strong or observant Jewish upbringing. As a child, she had attended Hebrew school two days a week and her family went to synagogue a few times a year, although she had not had a bat mitzvah. As an adult, her connection to Judaism had increased and she was a member of various Jewish organizations and educational groups; she was even considering studying to have a bat mitzvah as an adult. Judaism was now a very important part of her life:

> Yes, it's a vital part of who I am … *it's just absorbed into the blood stream* … just sort of part and parcel of who you are. You don't have to think about it, so it's just part of your identity. [emphasis added]

Similar to Ben, Jennifer did see her Jewishness as biological, yet this was also uncomfortable for her because of history:

> Yeah I think it is biological. Not only because … you're Jewish because your mother's Jewish but it is, it's passed down … I think we are a civilization, it's not just a religion, it's much more than that. *It's passed down by blood,* and it's based on a whole history, a whole civilization going back 2,000 years which gets just passed on through the generations … it is a religion but it's so much more, I don't know whether you'd call it a race, um … well some people did, didn't they? [emphasis added]

Nazi history and ideas about the biological difference of Jews make Jennifer uncomfortable about referring to Jews as a race, so much so that she avoids using the word Nazi and instead refers to 'some people'. At the same time, Judaism is passed down by blood and based on a 2,000 year shared history which makes it 'so much more' than just a religion. Jennifer described a recent trip to Italy:

> No matter what country you go to you'll find a similarity … in Florence we visited the synagogue there and looked around the museum and even there, I couldn't speak Italian and I was conversing with them in Hebrew and … it's just interesting that no matter where you go, there's a common language that you can use. And the links … I suppose you can sort of feel at home in shuls [synagogues] across the world really because there will always be that link.

Jennifer's connection to other Jews is a result of shared language, history and the 'links' that make her feel at home with other Jews throughout the world. Jennifer's description of Jewishness combines sentiments, blood, language, history and civilization – a mix of biological and social ideas that are so intertwined that they are neither one nor the other.

Daniel spoke explicitly about this sense of universal connection:

> You know I very rarely go to shul [synagogue] and you know my understanding of theology and spiritual things is so compromised and confused by my other knowledge now that I find it very hard to relate to the community ... the identity is really 'do you know me'? I recognize you ... and that's the comforting and positive thing. You know you go to Hong Kong or you know somewhere or other where two non-religious Jews nonetheless know each other because of the deep buried institutionalized parts of their identity which the rest of the time they ignore.

Daniel described his connection to other Jews as a 'recognition' that is comforting and transcends localities. Being Jewish unites Jews from all over the world who do not even know each other, and for Daniel this deep sense of connection is not a result of ritual observance. Rather, Daniel acknowledges that this recognition may be the result of 'institutionalized', rather than inborn, parts of identity. This is neither a religious nor a biological way of conceptualizing Jewishness.

Rebecca was an American woman in her late forties who had been living in London for the past 10 years. She was married, had no children and was a business professional working for a large American corporation. She had survived breast cancer and had a very strong family history, with her grandmother, great aunt, aunt and mother all having the disease. Her mother had died at the age of 53, when Rebecca was 23. Rebecca described her Jewish identity as a 'cultural identity'. Her family was 'very reformed' and she had had a secular upbringing, where Jewishness was more of a political identity associated with Israel. She did not have a bat mitzvah or attend synagogue while growing up and although her husband was not Jewish, she described feeling a 'definite bond' when she was with other Jewish people:

> I immediately just feel more understood, in a very kind of non-verbal way ... I just feel more myself, in a way ... even though ... I'm as ignorant of the Jewish religion in some ways as a lot of non-Jews but ... I think it is like shared rituals ... we just share more of that sort of history ... just growing up and ... knowing what it's like to sit at a table the first night of Seder [Passover meal] and being a little kid and just wanting to eat. Like we've all been there, and it's just an experience that you don't talk about, you would never talk to someone about that ... but you have them and other people don't have them.

Rebecca describes an unspoken understanding with other Jews and a sense of comfort that allows her to feel more herself. Rebecca feels more comfortable with other Jews because of the shared background and experiences that act as a common reference point. Rebecca's description of being a child during the Passover meal reminded me of my own childhood, and I understood exactly how Rebecca experienced the idea that as Jews (albeit Euro-American Jews) we had shared a similar upbringing. At the same time, Rebecca thought of her Jewishness biologically:

> I quite do think of my Jewishness in a biological way. Yeah I think I do. I think just in terms of how I think about, you know, like even just things like how I would change my physical self if I could. You know it would be like, the first thing would be like longer legs [laughter from us both] and you know when I'm with my Jewish friends like they all have kind of like stumpy legs like me right? [laughter] ... I can't think of one exception to that in my circle of Jewish friends. So that's what I mean by I think I do feel quite connected biologically.

Rebecca's 'biological' connection relates to her physical self and the trait she believes to be Jewish – 'stumpy legs'. She told me that she did not feel shame about this; in fact, she said (with a laugh): 'On the other hand I'm always the first one up a mountain right, like my legs are very, they're very functional which I appreciate so there's good sides as well.'

For Rebecca, the physical similarity only strengthened her sense of connection to other Jews. The idea of having Jewish physical traits arose in other interviews as well. People talked about their 'Jewish hair' or 'Jewish noses' and often used 'blond hair and blue eyes' as a shorthand way to refer to someone who was not Jewish. Physical similarities provide another boundary that demarcates Jews and were not shameful or problematic but contributed to a sense of sameness and shared characteristics that united Jews with one another. Even though physical appearance may appear to be a 'biological' boundary, it is also an incredibly 'social' practice. Glenn (2010) has traced the continuous and shifting public Jewish discourse about whether Jews 'look Jewish' and how Jews have attached complex and contradictory meanings to their looks. Real and imagined physical differences both mark Jews as stereotypically other and serve as symbols in a shared ethnic identity (Glenn 2010). According to Glenn (2010: 79), 'Jewish looks' have always had an important role in self-definition and 'for Jews ... Jewishness can be read on the body'. Now that Jews are primarily classed as 'White' and 'Euro-American', and many people who call themselves Jews have no affiliation or tangible connection to organized community life or institutions, naming and claiming of Jews by others on the basis of biological descent constitute a 'secular ritual that helps maintain a sense of uniqueness and historical connectedness among Jews' (Glenn 2010: 83). Thus 'looking for Jews is a fundamentally Jewish epistemology – a way of knowing ... who is Jewish' (Glenn and Sokoloff 2010: 8). It is also important to point out that my own role as a fellow Ashkenazi Jew created a safe environment in which individuals were able to make such comments about 'Jewish looks', and in fact sometimes individuals thought that I looked like a relative or someone they knew.

Sarah had grown up in the United States among many other Jewish families and as an adult she had lived in New York City, where approximately 13 per cent of the entire world Jewish population lives.[2] She did not believe in organized religion, yet this did not diminish her personal sense of being Jewish:

> I've always been an atheist, as long as I can remember, ever since I was six years old and started to think about it. And so I am not a religious person at all, and I don't like organized religion very much. On the other hand, I feel very Jewish, you know my identity is totally Jewish.

Most of the secular individuals interviewed expressed a similar feeling that their Jewish identity was not connected to religious observance or attendance at synagogue, but this did not mean that they did not still 'feel Jewish' and see themselves as such. This attitude was also reflected by the survey respondents; 10 per cent described themselves as religious/observant, 69.5 per cent as traditional/somewhat observant and 17 per cent as non-religious/secular. Respondents were also asked how strongly they identified with being Jewish, and 70 per cent said 'very strong'. As expected, all of the religious/observant respondents indicated that their Jewish identity was very strong; of the respondents who self-identified as non-religious/secular, nearly 50 per cent identified very strongly with their Jewish identity and the other 50 per cent moderately strongly.

Sarah was married to someone non-Jewish and they had one daughter. In describing her marriage, as well as the marriage of her non-Jewish friend to a German Jew, Sarah referred to the 'tangible' Jewish traits which could be inherited, or not, by children:

> The differences seem to me so built in ... one of my best friends is a you know nice girl from Nottingham who converted to Judaism, married a very clear German Jew ... and those little boys are, you know they look like my nephews. They look like little Jewish intellectual boys, whereas my daughter doesn't have that quality really. I mean do you know what I mean? For me it is a tangible quality ... I love to read you know but she doesn't. It doesn't mean she hasn't got the Jewish genes ... but there is that sort of intellectual quality that you recognize, also internalized, and she doesn't seem to be of that bent ... she looks like my mother in law ... she doesn't seem to have a great crying out to be identified as a Jew.

Yet, at the same time, when I asked Sarah about whether her daughter would identify herself as Jewish when she was an adult, she said: 'Those are issues much more of cultural identity issues. I am not sure they are so genetic.'

For Sarah, being, and seeming, Jewish are 'tangible' and 'built in' traits. They include 'Jewish genes', a certain type of intellect, a love of reading, and looking Jewish. Yet when asked about her own daughter's identity, she feels this is a 'cultural' rather than 'genetic' identity question. Teasing out what is biological and what cultural is impossible because her views express a conflation of culture and biology that cannot be disentangled.

David described his upbringing in South Africa as being not especially Jewish and 'almost rejectionist' because of his family's desperate need to be seen as English rather than Jewish in South Africa. Despite this lack of Jewish upbringing, he still always 'felt Jewish' and, following his father's death, when he was a teenager, he discovered a small booklet on how to practise Judaism at home, which stimulated his interest, and over the course of his life he had become very interested in Judaism. When he arrived in London as a young adult, he took Yiddish and Hebrew lessons and became involved with his local synagogue. Judaism had become such an important part of his life that he had spent the last four years compiling and writing a practical introduction to Judaism, which had recently been published. He hoped the book would inspire others to take up Judaism, just as the booklet he discovered as a teenager had done for him. For David, being Jewish was also about more than ritual observance:

> So for me, social action, social conscience, behaving in a way in which I would be proud of myself when I look in the mirror the last thing at night, is more important than whether I have a bacon sandwich or not [referring to the ritual of keeping kosher].

As a child, he was sent to an Anglican school where he was the only Jewish child and encountered anti-Semitism. At school he was referred to as the 'Jew boy'; being Jewish was 'a label that you put on yourself' and meant that 'we're a little bit different'. Political tensions around Israel also made David feel more comfortable around other Jews:

> I feel much more comfortable with people who if I mention the word Israel is [*sic*] not gonna look at me as the Christ killer or something like that. However nice and liberal and inclusive and everything else … I feel on edge … *one feels comfortable within the family.* [emphasis added]

David refers to other Jews as 'family' to describe the sense of safety and solidarity he feels with other Jews. Ben had also faced anti-Semitism growing up in France and being one of a small number of Jewish students at school. He also had very strong views regarding Israel, having travelled and lived there previously. Similar to David, he felt Israel could be a source of conflict and tension with non-Jews:

> I like spending time with Jews but you know it's not absolutely imperative for me by any means. I mean, most of my closest friends in the world it

so happens are Jewish. I make it clear early on that Israel's important to me and if that's a problem for you, we shouldn't have anything in common.

Both David and Ben referred to the political situation in Israel and how being with other Jews provided a sense of safety and comfort, free from anti-Semitism and tensions over Israel. Being Jewish could also be a source of pride and create a sense of being special. People mentioned the high number of Jewish individuals that had contributed to science, medicine, the arts, philosophy and various other domains as evidence that Jews were exceptional and had achieved great things. I often heard it mentioned that Jews have won more Nobel prizes than any other group.

When I first arrived at Daniel's house, he told me how he had always assumed Jews were genetically or biologically superior in terms of intelligence and had contributed so much intellectually to society. Daniel believed there was something special about being Jewish: 'So for example the Jews from the nineteenth century onwards have been fantastically rich participators and contributors in lots of areas. We should have pride in that ... the amazing achievers that we've been in the last 200 years.' For Michael, being Jewish made him feel special: 'That is cool because I have got this Jewish heritage, and ... that is pretty amazing. And Judaism, for me at least, it's that extra thing that makes me a little bit different which I embrace.'

We have seen that most individuals had multifaceted ways of identifying as Jewish. Being Jewish is a co-production of 'blood' and being born to a Jewish mother, as well as the shared history, rituals and language that coalesce to create a sense of solidarity and relatedness to Jews around the world. Yet these are neither clearly biological nor cultural notions and in fact the categories easily 'bleed' (metaphorically) into one another. Finkler (2000: 15) proposes that in all cultures kinship demarcates 'certain individuals by their significant same', and she distinguishes between those who experience themselves as a member of a significant same group and feel a sense of solidarity and relatedness because of shared experience, such as friends or co-religionists, and those who experience themselves as a member of a family or group who share DNA. She argues that shared experience, regardless of shared DNA material, is the basis of being in the world, interacting with others and feeling moral responsibility. Shared DNA does not require social interaction and as a result does not induce a sense of shared responsibility to those who are related to you. Yet in the above passages it is evident that Jews experience a sense of relatedness that is based on both shared blood and lineage and shared experience that is not reliant on physically growing up in the same household, as Finkler implies.

In the following sections I explore the ways in which genetic disease was interwoven with people's Jewish identity and whether genetic knowledge about disease did lead to a significant alteration in people's understanding of what being Jewish means.

Genetic disease: reiterating or altering connections

Jennifer was awaiting an appointment at her local genetics unit to discuss genetic testing. We were discussing the fact that the risk was higher for Ashkenazi Jews:

> It wouldn't make me not want to be an Ashkenazi Jewish woman because I've got a very strong sense of my identity and it's very important to me. So I guess I'm sort of like well that's how it is and that's how it was and we just have to live with it. And that's the history and that's you know how it came to be but um, yeah, but it wouldn't make me sort of not want to be who I am ... how does it feel knowing that I am at a greater risk? Yeah that's kind of unfortunate but then I look at all the positive wonderful stuff that I get out of it and I think well hey you weigh up the good and the bad together as you know, you do in all aspects of life.

For Jennifer, the benefits she derived from being Jewish far outweighed any drawbacks related to having an increased risk of disease. Jennifer's first cousin Anna had a similar view: 'No I mean my background isn't something that I can pick. Your family is rich with its own background and ... you know it's just one unfortunate aspect.'

When Elizabeth and I talked about the risk being greater because she was Ashkenazi Jewish, she told me: 'I always say I'm Jewish, that's pretty much what describes me. It's not Israel. It's not Ukrainian. It's not German ... it's Jewish and whatever comes with this whether it's breast cancer or whatever there is.'

Although David did not have a family history of disease, when we discussed genetic disease he said:

> I don't think you can define Jewishness by predisposition towards Tay-Sachs. No. I think that is just a little quirk in the background of what it means to be Jewish ... So I think 'I'm Jewish, I may have a gene or I may not but that's part of ... the package that I come with.' That's not defining my Judaism.

For the individuals described above, being at increased risk was simply one aspect of being Jewish that did not take away, on the whole, from the benefits derived from being Jewish, and some even described it as not relevant at all. Importantly, they all had positive experiences and derived personal fulfilment from being Jewish, and while genetic disease might be 'unfortunate', it did not radically alter, or negatively affect, the way they conceived of their Jewishness.

For Rebecca, her genetic risk actually reinforced her sense of connection with other Jews, and particularly other Jewish women. She was awaiting the results of her BRCA mutation test when we talked about the increased risk:

> I mean I liked the connection of that I think yeah … in terms of identity … I liked feeling that genetic connection to a group of people, yeah … I felt connected to history in a different sort of a way … kind of like a sense of being part of a bigger community, of women in particular.

Rebecca liked the idea that all Ashkenazi Jews are related biologically and described nostalgia for her childhood in the United States and the feeling of being 'part of that bigger family'. Since moving to London, she had had less exposure to other Jewish people and she missed that contact. In London she felt people were very 'ignorant' about Jews, and even highly educated British people often made 'snide comments about Jews' that she found 'really upsetting and really shocking'. She described being at a business meeting with a very-high powered person in her company who was unaware that it was the Jewish new year, or that there was a separate Jewish calendar. This experience stood in contrast to her experiences in New York where there is a very high Jewish population. Rebecca described a sense of alienation and not being understood by non-Jews, which is consistent with her earlier comment that she felt more understood and more herself around other Jews. A biological connection was appealing to Rebecca, who currently felt distanced from other Jews and the sense of community she had felt living in New York. We discussed an online *New York Times* video article chronicling a young healthy BRCA mutation carrier's decision to undergo a prophylactic mastectomy:[3]

> I felt identified with her … and her mother and all those women, those beautiful women and all that stuff. And so yeah, if I'm not part of that then it'll just be irritating … it'll be like 'how can I just be randomly unlucky?' … I guess in a way, if there's not a genetic link … yeah maybe it'll be a little disappointing.

Genetics provides a framework for understanding why Rebecca and so many women in her family had developed breast cancer as opposed to being just 'randomly unlucky'. For Rebecca, a genetic 'link' creates a sense of connection to her mother and family, other women and Jews in general, which fits well with her pre-existing notion that her Jewishness is biological, while also providing a causal explanation for the disease.

Lori was an American graduate student living and studying in London. She was in her mid-twenties and had lost her mother to breast cancer as a teenager. We met at the family history clinic to which she had been referred for advice about her own risk. While Lori was too young for genetic testing currently, she was advised it was something she could consider in future. I interviewed Lori one evening a few weeks after her clinical appointment. Lori had had a 'secular' upbringing and although she did attend Hebrew school for a couple of years as a child, Judaism was not particularly important to her. Her mother had been an atheist but her father was more ritually observant. When we discussed being Jewish, she said:

> I think Judaism in my life sort of functions more as a culture, or kind of a very vague sort of cultural background as opposed to spiritual religion or something you draw spiritual fulfilment from ... I think it's really just how someone's raised ... I don't think about it in terms of biology.

Lori does not describe feeling that her Judaism is biological, yet she went on to say: 'I think that these potential genetic mutations, Tay-Sachs disease, breast and ovarian cancer mutations, I mean that's what brings it back to a biological level obviously.'

For Daniel, genetic disease among Ashkenazi Jews helped to define them as a distinct group:

> I would have thought that if there are distinctive Jewish diseases then there must be distinctive Jewish genetic components. Now it may not be enough to found a whole identity, but ... it makes it quite difficult to resist the conclusion that if one was trying to define a group, meaning draw boundaries between it and another group, even if they weren't clear boundaries ... still it's an indicator!

Despite Daniel's acknowledgement that the boundaries would be unclear and porous when trying to define the group, it is hard for him to resist the conclusion that disease genes are an indicator that there are genetic aspects to being Jewish and this serves to reinforce the boundaries between Jews and non-Jews. For Lori and Daniel, disease genes demarcate Jews in some way and reiterate a boundary between Jews and non-Jews. In chapter two we saw that genetic disease and mutations can be used to infer Jewish origins in what Neulander (2006) calls 'disease-based Judaism'. In the above passages we can see that genetic disease does not lead to the creation of a new identity but rather reinforces the pre-existing boundaries or ways in which individual 'Jewish' identity was understood. This was not a challenging way of thinking about Jewish belonging and did not conflict with the other social and cultural ways in which they also experienced being Jewish.

In contrast, Rachel's story provides an example of how genetic knowledge about disease raised difficult questions about the biological basis of her own identity. Her sister was a BRCA1 mutation carrier and she had been referred to a clinic for a discussion about genetic testing. During her clinic appointment, Rachel explained that her sister had been tested for three specific genetic mutations and the genetic counsellor then mentioned that these were the three Ashkenazi founder mutations.[4] Rachel then told us that she had no idea the mutations had anything to do with being Ashkenazi Jewish. She was very surprised, and a conversation ensued between her and the genetic counsellor about why the mutations arose, and how other populations can also have an increased risk. After her appointment, Rachel told me that this added a whole new aspect to the myriad feelings she was already experiencing about whether or not to undergo genetic testing; when I interviewed her, we talked about this more fully. Rachel explained that Judaism did not play a big part in her daily life, as she was not ritually observant, and that mostly it was just a part of her background. Her upbringing was not particularly Jewish and so for Rachel:

> My experience of being Jewish was much more about being different and not the same. Yeah being different, so and kinda not something to identify strongly with ... although as I've gotten older then I can appreciate some of the nuances, and some of the comforting side of it is really nice.

Rachel's experience of Jewishness was primarily one of alienation, of being different from those around her, and not particularly something she felt connected to in a positive way. However, knowing that the risk was higher for Ashkenazi Jews raised some uncomfortable questions for her:

> The connection with Ashkenazi Jews is a very strange one only because ... then it brings you back to so it's in your genes. Is it in your genes? Is this a belief system that's being passed on or no? It's something that it's in your genes, that's kinda weird ... well because that brings it back to being a race maybe ... I think of it as a cultural identity ... which means there's a choice there ... and then suddenly it's like you have this because it came through this chain, because you come from this background.

For Rachel, the existence of genetic disease challenges her feeling that her Jewishness is a cultural identity as opposed to being inborn or 'in your genes'. Rachel thought of her Jewish identity as something that she had a choice about, as an identity that she could 'dip into' when it suited her; the implication that it was passed on genetically removed her ability to choose, which she did not like. Rachel was also struggling with the decision as to whether or not to undergo genetic testing, and she associated her risk with a sense that she did not have a choice about any of these things:

> It's kind of strange in that my conversation with you today ... it kept coming up that I kept talking about choices so obviously choice matters a lot to me ... but that has something to do with ... genes. The implication of things being carried through the genes not being about choices ... it's challenging your own ideas around your own sense of Judaism.

Amidst a strong feeling that she had no choice about her genetic risk, it was important to Rachel to feel her Judaism was under her control and something she did have a choice about; yet this was challenged by the implication that her genetic disease made her Jewishness biological. Rachel wondered whether perhaps because Judaism was not a big part of her life, the impact on her of having a genetic risk was greater than it might be for those whose Jewish identities were stronger.

Conclusion

This chapter began by describing the differing, and at times contradictory, ways in which Judaism defines belonging as a product both of upbringing and of being born Jewish. This complexity was reflected in the way people described their own Jewish identity and sense of belonging. Individuals described themselves as belonging to a cultural group brought together by shared history, upbringing, rituals and customs, which created a sense of connection and comfort with other Jews. At the same time, they conceived of Jewish belonging in biological terms, such as the requirement of having a Jewish mother, being born Jewish, having Jewish blood, and having Jewish physical traits. It is noteworthy that individuals did not use the word 'genetic' and only very occasionally used the word 'biological', but they did refer to birth and blood, which are arguably 'biological' in some sense. However, they simultaneously placed other things in the supposedly biological category, such as particular traits, characteristics, behaviours and appearances. Some discounted any biological basis to Jewishness, but this did not prevent them from making references to the requirement to have a Jewish mother, and Jewish 'blood'. Individuals experience not only Jewish identity but also the meaning of what is 'social' and 'biological' in multiple, complex and overlapping ways. This calls into question the very nature of both categories, as they appear to be indistinguishable. Thus while it is not new to suggest that the nature/culture opposition is problematic or often untenable (Franklin 1995, 2003, Goodman et al. 2003, Jasanoff 2004, Martin 1998, Rabinow 1996, Strathern 1992), this material beautifully illustrates the complexity and co-production of these categories. In particular, it highlights the multiple meanings of 'biological', which include ancestry, lineage, physical appearance, blood, Jewish mothers, genetic disease, lack of choice and many other things, which do not necessarily correspond to a biomedical genetic understanding of inheritance or genetics. Jewish mothers lead to Jewish children, but Jewish fathers do not. Being Jewish is concurrently a myriad other feelings, sentiments and experiences, such as shared history, culture and upbringing. Separating 'biological' concepts of identity from 'social' aspects is not feasible; nor is it an accurate reflection of what individuals experienced. On an individual level, people did not experience these conceptualizations as separate, distinct or in conflict with one another; instead they were so interwoven that it was not possible to separate what was biological and what was cultural, which were perfectly compatible ways of thinking about being Jewish.

The suggestion that genetics leads to a biologically essentialized view of identity (Azoulay 2003, Brodwin 2002, Kahn 2005) assumes one can separate the 'cultural' and 'biological' aspects of identity, or that identity is either one or the other, and fails to account for the ways in which biology can be an important part of Jewish identity that helps to define group belonging. Genetics does not necessarily cause Jewish individuals to re-orient themselves towards their kin in biogenetic terms (Finkler 2000, Novas and Rose 2000) because they already feel a sense of genetic relatedness towards not only their immediate families but Jews as a whole. Rather than a re-mapping or biologization of identity, this chapter shows how Jewish identity is already a combination of all these things, and yet none of these conceptions of being Jewish maps neatly onto categories of 'biological', 'genetic', 'social' or 'cultural'. However, Rachel's story provides an example of how genetic knowledge about disease can create an essentialist view of identity as inborn, natural and unalterable (Brodwin 2002: 326) and be interpreted as evidence that Jewishness is some kind of irreducible genetic category (Kahn 2005).

As regards the impact of genetic disease on Jewish identity, the individual experiences described here can be broadly divided into three categories (bearing in mind this is a sample of 19 individuals living in London). For those who had a positive or fulfilling experience of Judaism, genetic disease was simply one aspect of being Jewish that might be unfortunate but did not detract from the overall benefits they derived from being Jewish. For some women, such as Rebecca, genetic disease actually created a sense of connection to other Jews and reinforced her sense of belonging. It is worth noting that Rebecca expressed her longing for a connection with other Jews, and this biological relatedness may have helped fulfil that desire. Lastly, for Rachel the notion that her Jewishness might be biological was more problematic, and this may have been related to the fact that she did not experience Judaism in a positive way; rather, it was more of an alienating identity that made her feel different.

For most individuals, being at risk of genetic disease and the implication that one is part of a biological or genetic group were consistent with how they already perceived themselves. Biology, blood and genes are part of the vocabulary for Jews who see themselves as related to one another through shared blood and history. This supports Prainsack's (2007) finding that genetics can actually serve to reinforce notions of belonging among Jews because it fits with pre-existing notions of collectivity. In discussing the Israeli context, Prainsack (2007: 95) found that the concept of a Jewish population or biological genetic group is relatively unproblematic because it corresponds with 'established narratives' of belonging and serves to reinforce notions of 'groupness and collectivism'. Whereas population categories are highly problematic in some places, in Israel they serve an important political purpose of preserving the boundaries of existing collective identities and the distinction between Jews and non-Jews, which is important for the maintenance of the Israeli state. Kahn (2005) suggests that biological reasoning about Jewish belonging may be particularly appealing for those whose sense of Jewishness is not a result of commitment to the ritual laws and customs of Judaism, and interviewees repeatedly described their Jewishness as not being the product of ritual observance.

The following chapter continues to explore women's experiences of being at increased risk and specifically how genetic breast cancer and mutations could convey memories of the past (both individual and collective) yet also raise considerable anxiety for women.

5 History, memory and the BRCA genes

> Genetic inheritance establishes depth and continuity with previous generations and unifies people with their past.[1]
>
> (Finkler 2001: 249)

An ongoing theme throughout this book is the way in which genes provide connections to the past, origins and ancestors, and at the same time to the future and future generations. Jews have long-standing concerns with their origins and ancestry (Kahn 2005) and there are many ways genetics has been used to explore this past, as the Cohen modal haplotype and mitochondrial DNA studies described in chapter two demonstrated. This chapter begins by describing the interest many individuals had in recalling their ancestral past through constructing family trees and doing genealogy research in general. However, genealogy tracing serves another purpose for those with family histories of cancer, as it is necessary to assess women's risk in clinic. Genetic disease can bring individuals closer to their ancestors, especially as it involves recalling previous generations (Finkler 2000). For those with family histories of disease, the process of determining risk locates an individual within a 'network of relations' where it is necessary to recall family members from previous generations with disease, think of those family members currently living who will need to know about the risk, and future generations who may also be at risk (Novas and Rose 2000: 490). This process of remembering previous generations with breast cancer could also be accompanied by silence and lack of memory, something that appeared to be a result of the anxiety and worry that women faced about their own risk. Women had to confront the conflicting burdens and gifts that knowledge of genetic risk can create for them (Hallowell 1999, Kenen 1996).

Recollection through family trees

Genealogy tracing is a form of recollection that has become very popular in recent years (Finkler 2000, Nelson 2008, Obasogie 2009). Genealogy websites, both in general and specifically for Jews, have proliferated to help people trace their family histories. JewishGen is an umbrella website that helps

Jewish genealogists investigate their origins, with the explicit aim of ensuring Jewish continuity for present and future generations. It provides various resources, including numerous databases containing entries of towns and surnames to facilitate ancestral research. Over 75 Jewish genealogical societies exist throughout the world (including in the US, Canada, Argentina, Australia, Belgium, Brazil, Denmark, France, Germany, Great Britain, Israel, Netherlands, Russia, South Africa, Sweden, Switzerland and Venezuela) and since 1981 an annual conference on Jewish genealogy is held in a different city. I encountered numerous individuals who were looking back into the past by constructing family trees and doing genealogy research to discover more about their personal origins. Ben did not have a strong connection with being Jewish in terms of religious observance, but visiting Israel in his late teens significantly changed how he felt and made his Jewish identity very important to him. Ben described this first visit as a 'turning point' in his life:

> Going to Israel, you know, just seeing Israel, witnessing the country just gave me kind of factual reasons to justify to myself, align myself as a Jew ... the bottom line is that going to Israel made me understand that I am above, first and foremost a Hebrew ... I mean all these experiences were very intense and it really just felt like déjà vu – and just the basic feeling of arriving there ... All of a sudden I arrive at Ben Gurion airport and ... look to the left, look to the right, they're all Jewish! [laughter] ... and I just loved that.

Ben explained that he self-consciously chose to refer to himself as a Hebrew rather than a Jew because he believes that being Hebrew includes the non-religious aspects of being Jewish which he felt strongly connected to despite not practising ritual Judaism. Being surrounded by Jews was not something he had experienced growing up in a primarily non-Jewish environment and at a non-Jewish school in France, where he had at times encountered anti-Semitism. Arriving in Israel created a sense of déjà vu – a feeling as though he had been to Israel before. Brodwin (2002: 327) describes a similar experience undergone by American Jews who visit the Western Wall in Jerusalem and report that their collective history has suddenly become material, tangible and visible. On one of his visits to Israel Ben discovered the Museum of the Jewish Diaspora at Tel Aviv University, where there are facilities to help individuals trace their genealogy. He subsequently returned to do some research into his own family's origins:

> The closest I could get is finding out information about my family which dated back to 1820, of you know Latvian Lithuanian Jews and I would love to one day go over there just because I think that there's something very rewarding just to breathe the air of one's forefathers and foremothers and that's something that feels very special to me. It just seems like a way, a trip into the past which just makes *the whole concept of time collapse in*

a way. And you know, it's uh, it's something which can make me feel quite sentimental. [emphasis added]

Ben referred to time collapsing to explain how close doing genealogy research made him feel to his ancestors. Visiting Lithuania would allow him to 'breathe the air' of his ancestors and create a physical connection between him and his Lithuanian lineage:

> That's when I realized that it's a great privilege to be Jewish just because it's such a long history and it's something that should be upheld at all costs. There are so few of us ... I mean it's a blessing ... so I feel like looking back at the roots which are on record gave me a way of you know linking up with even more distant remote roots, of having ... nearly certainly been part of an existence in the very distant past in ancient Israel.

Genealogical research creates a sense of pride and belonging, while reinforcing Ben's connection not only to his own Lithuanian ancestors but also to the collective history of Jews in ancient Israel. His reference to there being 'so few of us' also expresses his demographic concerns about the decreasing population.

Jennifer felt a strong affinity to her family's Eastern European origins and described her mother's experience of visiting Russia:

> I'm third generation and yet it's funny I remember my mum saying she went back to Russia. They went on this holiday about nine or ten years ago and she wrote, I kept the postcard, and she said I feel at home. I thought how bizarre, my mum brought up in England but ... she actually felt quite, sort of, at home ... So you can be many generations on but there are certain things are just kind of very strong inside you.

Despite being born in England, Jennifer's mother carries an internalized connection to her historical roots and ancestral home in Russia.

David had been tracing his genealogy and collecting family history data for over 20 years and had created a website with all the information from his research. This comprehensive website contained details of the family tree, family history, the town in Lithuania where his family originated, maps, photographs and a page to contact David if you are part of the family. David explained his interest as being a way to learn more about himself and who he was: 'Sometimes in order to know where you are going you have to know where you have come from. That's where the mission started. Where am I? Who am I? Why am I what I am?'

The website had allowed David to find out whether other individuals with the same last name as him were indeed part of the same family. According to him, when Jews arrived in South Africa from Eastern and Central Europe, they would sometimes change their name or hide their identity, which meant that some individuals who carried the same surname as David might not be

'genuine'. David and one of his distant relatives with the same surname underwent genetic testing on the Y chromosome to see if they were in fact related to
one another. The genetic test revealed that they were probably not related but,
as David pointed out, this did not answer the important question of 'who is the
real one'. Another consequence of his online genealogy was that a family
member had contacted him about a genetic disease her child suffered from and
to investigate if any other family members had this disease. David described using
the website to contact other relatives to inquire about this particular disease
but there were no other cases in the family. Similar to Ben, David's family
history tracing was a project that he pursued for his own interest and to learn
more about himself rather than for the purpose of learning about diseases.

Other individuals also described doing genealogy research. Mira's son was
in the process of compiling a family tree and was discovering things that she
had not known about her own family, such as their German origins. Lori told
me that since childhood she had always wanted to know which countries her
grandparents came from but that this could not be pinned down. Rebecca
wanted to go back to Romania where her grandparents were born to reconnect
with her past. When she and her husband had been considering adopting a
child, she had wanted the baby to be from Romania because of the connection
she felt through her grandparents. Nancy, on the other hand, was a woman
who knew very little about her family tree but told me that this was 'a shame
actually' and that she hoped to find out more one day in the future. When
Nancy and I discussed both having relatives who had emigrated from Eastern
Europe to America, she made a joke that 'our relatives probably knew each
other'. When Sarah and I discussed where in Eastern Europe our ancestors
came from, she said we were surely 'from the same places'. Family history and
genealogy tracing constitute 'repositories of communal and social memory'
(Finkler 2000: 10) of the shared past and ancestors of Ashkenazi Jews, while
also reaffirming the interrelatedness of Jews.

In some cases, genealogy tracing also helped to map out the incidence of
cancers in the family, as in Susan, Jennifer and Anna's family. Susan and
Anna were sisters who were awaiting their results following BRCA mutation
testing, and Jennifer was their first cousin. When I arrived to interview Jennifer
in her home one afternoon, the first thing she showed me was an enormous
family tree. She unrolled a series of A4 sheets of paper that were taped together
and nearly went the entire length of her living room. The sheets contained a
computer-generated family tree with colour coded boxes identifying all the
maternal relatives she and her cousin Anna had traced so far, including those
from England, the USA, Denmark, France and Israel. Initially this project
had not been to trace diseases but simply arose because Jennifer and Anna had
an interest in genealogy dating back to childhood. However, once they began
to uncover the family history of breast cancer, the family tree had taken on
another purpose. Jennifer and I examined the family tree together and she
pointed out the relatives who had died of breast cancer, those who were
having screening, those who had had biopsies and those who were having

genetic testing. A separate document had been created by Anna that listed the names, relationships and types of cancer of all those who had been affected. I was amazed at the size and detail of the pedigree itself:

JM: Well this is amazing. I guess it's not very cheery but it came in a lot of use when you had to ...

JENNIFER: Start to work out patterns actually and I hadn't even thought about that but there are patterns. Just you know every branch, every sister or wherever there's been a sister who died of it, yeah, look at that, *it's gone down the branch.* [emphasis added]

Laura was also working on a 'family log project' to document the incidences of cancer in her own family. Laura and another relative who had breast cancer decided to create a family log as a way to record the past and help future generations:

I wanted to run this project with my mother's family about cancer in the family because I thought it was very important when I heard about this Ashkenazi woman BRCA1 BRCA2. I thought for us to have a family log, *for what's gone before, for the girls coming after,* and also the men ... well it was an idea to just mark down in a family tree-like way every single branch of the family ... and circulate it to everybody because sooner or later it's gonna help a doctor somewhere and one of the family somewhere along the lines. [emphasis added]

Laura believed the log was something that should be used by all Ashkenazi families:

Some people don't want to know, I can't believe it because it's not just about them. Even though I've got no birth children, I've got cousins and they've got children. Even on my dad's side and they've got daughters and sons and it's for them as well. It's not just for our families, it's for other families. So I think it's something that should unite us, not divide us ... I would like to start campaigning for people to have a family log, because I think it's so important.

While Laura has no children, and therefore no risk of directly passing on a mutation, she feels an obligation to her extended family. She also expresses a responsibility beyond her own immediate family to all Jewish families. Breast cancer is a community-wide issue and remembering past relatives with cancer is a mechanism to avoid disease in future generations. She explicitly states that people who choose not to find out about their family history are doing a disservice to all Jews, which again shows how disease becomes associated with the entire 'community' of Jews. Family logs and trees are ways of articulating history and ensuring that things are remembered and not forgotten.

Forgetting

In contrast, family histories and genetic risk could also be associated with a tendency to forget. Women claimed to forget details of their own breast cancer, their genetic testing status and various other aspects related to breast cancer in the family. I am using the word forget to encompass more than just mere forgetting but also to include a more complex lack of remembering or not acknowledging, and perhaps even avoidance of, some of the stressful aspects of being at increased risk. There were two reasons why I initially noticed this tendency to forget. First, sometimes women would claim to have forgotten and then go on to demonstrate quite a lot of knowledge about the things they could not remember. Second, I was surprised by women's claims of forgetting as these women did not strike me as the kind of women who forgot. Many of the women I interviewed were highly educated professional women, some of whom were very successful in their professions. There appeared to be a discrepancy between these women's daily achievements and accomplishments and their claims that they forgot so much about their disease or family history. While they sometimes reported being just too busy or distracted, I suspected that there might also be a more purposeful forgetting at work. I acknowledge that, as a researcher, it is impossible for me to know if women really did forget and I can only speculate based on the information they gave me, and my own interpretation of the material, whether or not this forgetting was significant. However, the forgetting, or rather lack of remembering, often appeared to be related to anxiety and worry.

High-risk women face various difficult issues and choices. For those who have not had breast cancer, there is the ongoing possibility that they are going to develop it in the future just as someone in their family did, frequently their mothers or sisters whom they had witnessed develop and sometimes die of the disease. For these women, screening was an important mechanism to detect and prevent getting breast cancer. However, the screening appointments themselves could raise anxiety and concern both in the days leading up to them and in the days following them while women waited for the results. As with all screening procedures, there is a risk of a false positive, in which case a woman is recalled for a second mammogram or screening procedure which then turns out to produce a benign result. This recall can cause considerable worry for the woman, who may think she has cancer while she awaits the second test and result.

During clinical consultations women frequently raised questions about the efficacy of mammography, notably if it will detect breast cancer early enough, how often it should be performed and at what age screening should begin. In addition, all the women I met had to deal with the possibility that they themselves might be BRCA mutation carriers. I met a variety of women, some who had undergone genetic testing, some who were awaiting results and others who had not decided if they wanted to be tested; yet in all of these cases there remained the possibility that women might be carriers. Even when the test result had been negative, if there was a strong family history, women were told there might be another gene or mutation that had simply not been discovered yet and so they remained in the high-risk category. In fact, 75 per cent of those with family histories are not found to have BRCA mutations, and no 'standard' approach exists to manage women with a family history and negative BRCA test (Ziogas et al. 2011).

For those who are found to be carriers, a whole host of other preventive strategies (including prophylactic surgery) have to be considered, which can be especially difficult as these options may come with significant behavioural and adverse psychosocial effects (Ziogas et al. 2011). Prophylactic surgery was very difficult for many women to consider, yet the efficacy of screening, which is the only alternative to surgery, could be an additional source of worry that made many women feel prophylactic surgery was the only (or best) option. Some women were more concerned about the increased risk of ovarian cancer, and the difficulty of detecting it, than their risk of breast cancer, which they felt could be more easily monitored and treated. Women with children also had to consider the implications for their own children. Thus, there were many upsetting and difficult issues that being at risk of genetic breast cancer raised for women.

There is no absolutely reliable method of early diagnosis and prophylactic surgery does not entirely eliminate risk either, so that being a BRCA gene carrier can leave women with a lifelong fear and feeling of being a 'genetic time bomb' (Mor and Oberle 2008: 516). Finkler (2001) refers to those who are at increased risk of genetic disease as 'perpetual patients' because even those who are currently disease free or healthy can always potentially become ill as a result of their family history. 'Perpetual patients' have to attend regular screening and surveillance appointments or undergo prophylactic surgery despite not actually having the disease. People may become incessantly worried and begin to think in terms of 'when I get breast cancer' rather than 'if I get breast cancer' (Finkler 2001: 244).

Rebecca had been diagnosed with breast cancer the year before we met and successfully treated. When we met, she had already undergone a BRCA test for the Ashkenazi founder mutations but no mutation had been found. Her blood had then been sent off for a full screen (of the entire sequence of BRCA1 and BRCA2) but she had not yet received the results. She had a strong family history and her mother had died of breast cancer when Rebecca was 23. Her older sister had an early form of breast cancer and had been tested in the United States, but again no mutation had been found. Rebecca was expecting her test result to be negative:

> I don't know, it's very unscientific but I think I just assumed because my older sister was negative I just wasn't expecting it to be positive. Also because I think within that interview with the geneticist, or whatever it's called, the more she spoke to me, the more I realized that it could just be one of those flukes of things, you know, that a certain number of women at a certain point in their life are gonna have breast cancer.

The fact that her sister had tested negative gave Rebecca a sense that she too would be negative, despite the fact that she and her sisters all had an equal probability (50/50) of inheriting a mutation if there was one in the family. Rebecca may also have picked up on her genetic counsellor's ambivalence about the value and utility of genetic testing. In my experience, clinicians and genetic counsellors sometimes expressed ambivalence about the utility of the test, especially when many results came back as inconclusive or with no mutation found. On the last occasion when I saw Rebecca she was very upset by the news she had just received that her younger sister had also been diagnosed with breast cancer. We were in clinic and the genetic counsellor confirmed that no genetic mutation had been found when Rebecca's blood was tested for the second time. During our interview I asked Rebecca about her own diagnosis: 'Um, I should have brought it written down, this is how bad I am about it, it's just because I just don't keep these things in my head, um, there's four stages right?'

Rebecca's inability to remember the details of her own diagnosis 12 months earlier struck me as very out of character. Throughout the interview she minimized the impact of her breast cancer and her concerns about it being genetic. She was having regular screening and being followed up by her oncologist, which made her feel that there was nothing to worry about and that it was 'not a big deal'. Rebecca could see no reason why her surgeon was so insistent that she continue to be monitored annually; this is in fact routine clinical practice because there is always a possibility of recurrence. This view appeared to be more a result of Rebecca not wanting to be reminded of the possibility of a recurrence each time she attended a follow-up appointment. When describing her first appointment at the genetics unit, she recounted being surprised that talking about her mother's breast cancer had made her feel upset. Near the end of the interview Rebecca mentioned the scars on her breast from the surgery, and this was the first indication she gave that her experience of breast cancer had been difficult: 'It's just that I have this scar, and it's fine, it's a beautiful result and everything but sometimes when I look at the scar I'm like I wouldn't be so eager to do that again, for sure.' Rebecca seems to be trying to convince both of us that everything is fine, yet her scar acts as a physical reminder of something very difficult that she would not want to go through again. I had the sense that Rebecca's cancer, and the loss of her mother, had had a very large impact on her despite her attempts to minimize them.

Mrs Bernstein was an ultra-Orthodox Jewish woman whom I met when she was attending the family history clinic for her annual mammogram. Mrs Bernstein was interested in taking part in the research, but when I entered the clinical consultation room I found her to be very tearful and upset. She explained that she always became emotional when she came to the clinic for her breast screening appointments. After I described the study, Mrs Bernstein told me she had no idea there was an increased risk of breast cancer for Ashkenazi Jews. I was initially surprised because she attended the family history clinic annually for breast screening and yet reported to have no idea that her increased risk was related to being Ashkenazi Jewish. In the end she decided not to take part as she felt it would be too upsetting for her. Later I informed the family history nurse about what had happened, and she told me that it was highly unlikely Mrs Bernstein would not have been informed about the risk for Ashkenazi Jews as she had attended an appointment with her specifically to discuss her family history and genetic testing. She went back to check the notes of their first consultation and, although she had not made a specific note in the patient's file, she told me it was almost impossible that the increased risk for Ashkenazi Jews would not have been mentioned at their first consultation, especially as Mrs Bernstein was ultra-Orthodox Jewish with ten children, one of whom had a genetic disorder. Mrs Bernstein found attending her annual screening appointment so stressful that it led her to tears and not recalling her increased risk as an Ashkenazi Jewish woman may have been a way of psychologically managing her high levels of anxiety.

Nancy also told me she had completely forgotten about the connection to being Ashkenazi Jewish until she received the information about my study: 'But I just remember knowing about that and forgetting until I went last week and they said you were doing this and I said "oh god yeah, now I remember".'[2] Rachel was another woman whose forgetfulness was mixed with anxiety over whether to undergo genetic testing. Rachel's sister was a BRCA1 mutation carrier with breast cancer, and she had a history of breast cancer on her paternal side of the family. When she arrived for her clinic appointment, she immediately told the genetic counsellor that, despite being aware of the possible risk for a long time, it had just hit her and she was feeling 'suddenly very emotional' and overwhelmed. It appeared that Rachel had pushed aside her worries and was surprised that she was finding all the issues she was facing regarding screening and genetic testing so upsetting. She had recently been through a battery of appointments to organize ovarian and breast screening and had just returned from a trip home to America, where she had visited her sister for the first time since she had been diagnosed with breast cancer, and who was undergoing chemotherapy. After the clinic appointment, I wrote in my own field notes that Rachel's surprise at suddenly feeling upset reminded me of all the other instances of forgetting combined with anxiety that I was encountering. Rachel was very knowledgeable and had a lot of information regarding the benefits and drawbacks of testing, screening and surgery. She had so many questions that the clinic appointment took an hour, which was double the usual allotted time.

After the appointment Rachel reiterated to me that she was feeling stressed and waiting for this appointment had made her very anxious. As she took an aspirin, she told me that being stressed caused her to forget things. Rachel expressed a great deal of conflict over whether to have the test or not. She felt pressure from her family, especially her mother, to have the test, while her sister was choosing to undergo prophylactic mastectomy and oophorectomy, which Rachel found very difficult to accept. She referred to these procedures as mutilating the body and could not imagine doing this herself. I had been very affected by Rachel's predicament and was relieved the genetic counsellor had reassured her that she did not have to rush into making a decision about undergoing testing. Rachel was advised to take as much time as she needed, and told that at any time she could ring up and arrange for another appointment and testing could be done quickly and easily because there was already a known mutation in the family. When I subsequently interviewed Rachel, she talked in more detail about the difficulties she was having accepting that she might not want to have the test.

> It is a matter of too much information and not enough at the same time, which is what makes it difficult, you know if we could do something really positive with the information but at the time where we're at, in some ways we know more than is helpful.

For Rachel, BRCA mutation testing produced both too much and not enough information at the same time. Given the limited and invasive management options, which Rachel was strongly opposed to, this was an accurate reflection of the predicament she was facing.

Rachel insisted that she was not that worried about her risk or the possibility of being a carrier:

> I'm not worrying about it ... if I was worrying about it, I would do it. I'm not worrying about it. I'm more worried about worrying about it if I were to find out that I also carry that gene. You know whether that's a state of denial or just a state of positive thinking ... who knows? I'm not gonna look for trouble ... I'm just concerned about how deep that could sink into my psyche if I were to find out that, in terms of it's just a predisposition, but [a] high rate risk one ... I'm not sitting here every day worrying about it at all! I'm not worrying, no I don't think I am.

Rachel repeatedly raised the possibility of being in 'denial' and even asked me whether I thought she was in denial. 'But then I know there are such things as denial, but I don't know if that's, how do you know if you're in denial over something?'

Despite her claims to the contrary, Rachel appeared to be quite anxious. She believed that knowing she was a carrier could cause her to worry more and possibly lead her to get cancer. Rachel was especially concerned about the risk of ovarian cancer and the lack of screening methods to detect it. The inability to see or feel the ovaries, as opposed to the breasts, led Rachel to feel vulnerable, and she had previously had two abortions and felt particularly protective about this area of her body. If she was a BRCA mutation carrier, she would want to have her ovaries removed to allay her anxieties about getting ovarian cancer and she wondered if she was avoiding facing this issue, especially as she viewed surgical removal of the breasts or ovaries as 'mutilation' which went against her 'feminist streak of body politics' and her feeling that prophylactic surgery came from a 'male dominated place': 'I believe in prevention but chopping off parts of the body, I'm not sure ... so by not knowing though, that's a different way to get rid of the worry I guess.'

At the same time, Rachel felt an obligation to have the test simply because the information was available:

> I'm definitely feeling pressured but there is also a part of me that feels like if that information is available which it didn't used to be then ... I still think though that if I'm doing the test it's because I would consider removing my ovaries as a prevention. Maybe it's just a lot of not wanting to deal with that! [laughter]

Hallowell (1999) describes how high-risk women may relinquish their right not to know about their genetic risk because of a perceived responsibility and obligation to manage their risk. In her discussion of prenatal screening, Kenen (1996) refers to the 'gift of knowing' as the belief that knowledge is intrinsically good, enabling patients to make more informed decisions, which may not always be the case.

Rachel saw her lack of physical and emotional resemblance to her family members with cancer, and the similarity of her breasts to those of her mother, who did not have breast cancer, as offering a protective mechanism:

> I'm sure it's not the least bit scientific but my body type ... is different, and if you look at my sister she is more similar to my aunt in that way, in their build, they're small, they're petite, but what that has to do with anything I don't know but there's that which could be genetic.

Rachel also referred to the similar emotional traits of her sister and aunt, both BRCA mutation carriers:

> And then there's their emotional make-up in some ways more similar ... in that they aren't so great at expressing, they're good at repressing emotion, and um my aunt certainly has a huge amount of anger and my sister ... she is more likely to push things down and also to ... put other people's needs before her own. And it just depends on whether you believe in any of these things ... For those reasons I'm not like, I'm a bit different from them both physically and emotionally.

According to Sontag (1990), cancer has frequently been characterized as a disease that results from repression of feeling. Sontag (1990: 100) refers to this as a 'fiction of responsibility' where emotional and character traits predispose individuals to cancer, especially repressed anger or sexual feelings. Family members who are trying to make sense of the patterns of inheritance of a disease may use the idea of certain traits that may predispose them to or protect them against inheriting the disease, and these understandings could be a psychological strategy to help individuals understand what is happening and feel protected (Richards 1996).

Sarah also described herself as being forgetful and having a terrible memory. One of the first things Sarah mentioned to me when I arrived at her house was that she was feeling particularly anxious about a recurrence. She was taking Tamoxifen prophylactically but was unsure how to differentiate the side effects of the drug, such as aching bones, from the signs that her disease had returned. Before she was diagnosed, and despite having two sisters with breast cancer, she had skipped two annual mammograms. She attributed this to being distracted but then acknowledged that it was 'craziness' for someone in her situation to miss two mammograms. I had encountered so much forgetfulness and/or lack of remembering that I enquired directly about it:

JM: But do you think it was almost purposeful or were you really just distracted and not thinking about it?
SARAH: [pause] I'm sure it was you know five parts denial and five parts this being convinced.

Sarah was convinced that she would not get breast cancer because she had read so many articles about dietary measures that helped to prevent cancer, such as drinking tea and eating broccoli, both of which she did. Women held multiple explanations and theories about why they may or may not be at increased risk of getting breast cancer, and these co-existed with their understanding that the breast cancer could be familial and passed down by a faulty gene. Their narratives combined genetic, environmental, psychological and lifestyle explanations as to the causation of their disease. Unfortunately, Sarah had developed breast cancer, just like her two other sisters. Sarah's attitude had completely changed as she was now convinced that her breast cancer was genetic, despite the fact that she had undergone testing and no mutation had been found.

Forgetfulness could also be associated with a denial or masking of the reality of the family situation. Michelle's mother had been treated for breast cancer five years earlier and Michelle had subsequently been seen at a genetics unit in a London hospital about the possibility of having genetic testing but had not taken any further action since then. As Michelle's mother had breast cancer, it was her mother who would have to be tested first to see if she was a mutation carrier, before Michelle could be tested. This is standard clinical genetic testing practice in the UK as the first person to be tested in a family must be an affected relative; this is the only way to definitively determine that the gene mutation is linked with the specific incidence of breast cancer. I probed into Michelle's decision and she then explained that her mother had not attended the genetics appointment with her. I asked if her mother was unwilling to have genetic testing and Michelle claimed that her mother had no problem with having the test but that they had just not 'got around to it'.

There appeared to be a discrepancy in Michelle's story as she described her genetics appointment:

> My mum wouldn't come with me. She's very strange my mother, but my dad came with me actually … the conclusion that they came to actually was that you know if my mum was just willing to have a blood test, they would check that for the gene and then you know obviously if it wasn't there then I wouldn't have it and then my daughter wouldn't have it either. I mean obviously if she did have it, then I would have to be tested and so would my daughter … but we haven't done it and we should do. We're very naughty 'cuz it's only a blood test.

Despite Michelle's claim that her mother was willing to have the blood test, it was Michelle, not her mother, who had sought the initial referral to the genetics unit, and this also indicated to me that Michelle, not her mother, was interested in testing. Michelle told me that her mother's first reaction upon being diagnosed was: 'what about my daughter because she's just had a daughter?'. I wondered whether Michelle's mother might have felt guilt about possibly being a carrier and passing on a mutation and, as a result, may not have wanted to have the test. Michelle minimizes the importance of the test by referring to it as a simple blood test that the family have just not managed to get done; however, it is potentially much more than a blood test as there are many implications of being a carrier for both Michelle and her family, especially as she had a very young daughter who could also be at risk. The idea that the family had just not got around to it was part of a larger theme of forgetfulness that arose repeatedly. Michelle had asked her GP about her own risk after what she described as a long period of forgetting to mention that her mother had been diagnosed with breast cancer.

MICHELLE: I then went to see my doctor, I kept on *forgetting* to tell my doctor that my mum had had breast cancer, and I … went to see her about something else and I said oh, by the way, my mum had breast cancer 5 years ago. Oh, she said, okay, I'll stop you there and we'll refer you up to the Hospital X.
JM: So it was a bit after your mum had had [breast cancer]?
MICHELLE: Yeah, purely because *I kept forgetting*. No other reason. [emphasis added]

I asked Michelle what advice the genetics unit had given her about her own risk and she told me she 'could not remember'. We discussed breast self-exam and again Michelle told me that she forgets to do it. However, when Michelle spoke about her mother's breast cancer or her own breast screening, she was very knowledgeable. She described accurately to me the length and type of treatment her mother had. She was familiar with the breast screening guidelines under the NHS and was planning on starting mammograms early by going privately when she turned 40 the following year. It appeared that her forgetting was not accidental but more symbolic of the fact that she did not actually want to acknowledge the potential risk that she felt about getting breast cancer, especially as she had two young children. She related a story to me about a recent cancer scare she had where lumps were found on her liver, which turned out to be benign. Michelle was unable to speak for an entire week while she waited for the results. She told me that if it had turned out to be cancer, she would have flown around the world to seek treatment as she would not allow her children to grow up without a mother. Michelle's story about her liver cancer scare reflected a much more concerned and anxious attitude about the possibility of getting cancer than the laissez-faire and forgetful attitude that she presented about genetic testing and her risk of breast cancer. Her insistence that the family had just not got around to having the blood test appeared to be masking a lot of worry as well as the possibility that her mother may not have wanted to have the test.

Sarah also described how one of her sisters had refused to have genetic testing:

> My youngest sister would not be tested. She was very much in denial about the whole thing. She was the one who died. Then my middle sister, she was married to a doctor at Hospital X too. My middle sister and my older sister both went to be tested after my middle sister was diagnosed, and I think my mother went too.

Sarah and Michelle both describe being forgetful and having bad memories, which leads them to forget to attend mammograms, do breast self-exam or tell their doctor about their family history, yet they also expressed considerable anxiety about the possibility of developing or having a recurrence of breast cancer. Each had a family member who did not want to have genetic testing. While Sarah attributes her sister's refusal to denial and an inability to deal with her own breast cancer, Michelle was insistent that the family had just not got around to it. It is not possible to know why Michelle's family had not undergone testing, but I had heard stories anecdotally and read about cases where parents felt guilt about being carriers and the possibility of passing a genetic mutation to their children. Rachel also described how her aunt, who was a BRCA mutation carrier, began acting 'weird' when her sister developed breast cancer, which Rachel attributed to her aunt's feelings of guilt. Gessen (2008) also found evidence of feelings of guilt among families where there is a BRCA mutation.

The above examples demonstrate the different ways in which forgetfulness was mixed with women's worries and anxieties about being at risk of genetic breast cancer, and in the following section I will explore more overt forms of secrecy and denial about family histories of breast cancer.

Cancer: historical shame and silence

Cancer has historically been associated with silence, shame and extreme fear because it has been regarded as a horrible disease that inevitably leads to death, with no redeeming virtue (Clow 2001, Press et al. 1997). It is the 'quintessential feared illness of the 20th century' (Press et al. 1997: 142) because it is seen as leading to a slow, agonizing, disfiguring and costly death, especially when treatment has historically been radical, invasive and often very traumatic for patients. Sontag (1990) argues that cancer patients have suffered in silence as a result of the stigma and shame attached to the disease, particularly because of a pre-war tendency to blame patients for the onset of cancer. Clow (2001) claims that this silence was not specific to cancer but was rather a product of a general reticence to talk about disease in the context of a culture that valued privacy in matters of illness and dying.

Proctor (1999) has specifically examined the relationship between the Nazis and cancer. According to Proctor (1999), cancer has always been a frustrating disease because of its insidious growth and notorious resistance to therapeutic intervention. In the 1920s and 1930s, cancer incidence was on the rise and it was a 'difficult symbol: a disease of civilization, of modernity, a not yet conquered foe' (Proctor 1999: 8). Cancer became a metaphor for all that was seen to be wrong with society, and not just in Germany. The language used by Nazis in connection with cancer included describing tumours as Jews and Jews as tumours, and cancer became synonymous with malevolence and malignance (Proctor 1999).[3]

Denial and late diagnosis

One consequence of the shame and stigma surrounding cancer is that people can be reluctant to acknowledge their symptoms or illness because they see it as equivalent to a death sentence (Sontag 1990). As a result, they seek treatment only at a very late stage, when the disease is no longer treatable. Successful treatment for breast cancer and long-term survival are directly related to the point at which it is detected. The earlier the stage at which breast cancer is diagnosed, the more successful the treatment is likely to be. Some women I met, or members of their family, reported not seeking advice until a very late stage. Between 2004 and 2007 a well-known British journalist named Dina Rabinovitch wrote about her experience of breast cancer in a series for the *Guardian* newspaper. Her Jewish identity and religious life figured heavily in her writing, which was eventually published as a book that was launched at Jewish Book Week in February 2007 (Rabinovitch 2007). Many women followed Dina's column and story, including some of the women I interviewed. One significant aspect of Dina's story was that she had a growing lump in her breast for over three years before she went to her doctor. Dina attributed her lack of action to a certainty that she was not at risk of breast cancer because she had children at a young age and breastfed each child for over a year, factors known to decrease the risk of breast cancer but certainly not to prevent it from occurring. Just as Sarah thought dietary measures such as tea drinking protected her, Dina thought she was safe from getting breast cancer because of her childbearing. Dina also claimed not to have known about mammograms, and some of the women I interviewed were very sceptical of how a smart and worldly woman such as Dina could not know about mammograms or could think that a growing lump was nothing to worry about. In her book she acknowledges that there is a seeming discrepancy between her educational/ professional background and her dismissal of her potential risk of breast cancer (Rabinovitch 2007).

Rebecca also recounted how her mother had a massive lump in her breast before she sought medical advice and how she was unsure whether this was because her mother was simply unaware that the lump could be a risk or because she chose to ignore it. She suggested that perhaps her mother's unconcerned attitude was due to a generational difference and a lack of knowledge about breast cancer. Yet, Rebecca's great aunt and grandmother also had breast cancer, so it was difficult for her to believe her mother would not have been conscious of her risk:

> I was thinking about my mother, only in terms of my own diagnosis ... because by the time ... she diagnosed herself there was like a massive lump in her breast ... I don't know what the answer is, it's either she was unaware that there might be an increased risk or was aware and just chose to ignore it which I can understand as well. I don't know which it is, but it surprised me because she was quite a kind of controlling, you know, she took care of things. She wouldn't have necessarily let something slip like that.

Rebecca suspects that perhaps her mother made a conscious decision on some level not to acknowledge her own risk of breast cancer. She believed that levels of awareness and the quality of treatments were so much higher today than they were in her mother's time, which may help to explain why her own mother did not survive. She mentioned a friend's mother who had recently been diagnosed and successfully treated as evidence that treatments and knowledge about breast cancer had advanced so much since her mother's treatment: 'Which I guess just shows in a generation how information has changed so dramatically.'

When people described the history of cancer in their families, they often mentioned that cancer was not talked about or discussed, especially in previous generations. This lack of historical information about cancer is something I encountered frequently in my professional experience, especially when women were trying to obtain details of their family history. Often there are no medical records available that detail the exact diagnoses of relatives' cancers in previous generations, and women often reported a general reluctance of older relatives to discuss cancer in the family, especially women's cancers such as breast or gynaecological cancers. Press et al. (1997: 144) claim that in the early twentieth century women's breast and reproductive cancers were the most frequently diagnosed cancers and that cancer was seen as a woman's disease, and that this perceived link between cancer and women may have contributed to the impression that cancer was especially private and shameful. For some Ashkenazi Jews, the destruction of family records or the loss of previous generations as a result of the Holocaust exacerbates the difficulties of family history tracing. Sharsheret, the American Jewish breast cancer support organization (described in chapter two), devoted an entire symposium to the role of the Holocaust in breast cancer families, and described the difficulty of family history tracing in situations where many relatives were lost in the Holocaust.

Lori's mother became ill when Lori was 9 years old and had died when she was 15. We first met at her clinic appointment, where she was feeling very anxious about her risk and was nearly impossible to reassure. Lori's mother had two primary breast cancers (considered the equivalent of two separate diagnoses) below the age of 40 and while this was the only family history, Lori's risk was still elevated. Genetic testing was not recommended as the risk of breast cancer was extremely low for a woman below 30, and Lori was still in her mid-twenties. In addition, mammography is not particularly effective in younger women and so little could be done in terms of screening until Lori was at least 30 years of age. During the consultation the family history nurse explained the drawbacks of having genetic testing at this stage because there would be so little benefit. Unsurprisingly, the lack of available options did not help to alleviate Lori's anxiety. Lori believed that the BRCA genes could 'spontaneously mutate' and was extremely concerned that, even though her mother was the only family member to have had breast cancer, she too could suffer a spontaneous mutation and get the disease. The genes do not spontaneously mutate but are usually a result of historical founder mutations that are passed down from parent to child, and Lori was somewhat relieved when the genetic counsellor explained this. Lori's aunt, her mother's sister, was alive and well in her fifties. If there was a mutation in the family, then both Lori and her aunt had an equal probability (50 per cent) of carrying the mutated gene. The fact that her aunt had not developed breast cancer was further evidence that there might not be a mutation in the family. Lori remained convinced that she was more at risk than her aunt despite the family history nurse telling her otherwise. In fact, Lori told me she was certain she was going to be a BRCA mutation carrier and develop breast cancer:

> I felt certain that I would test positive ... I do sometimes feel like deep inside I believe that someday I am going to be diagnosed with cancer ... unfortunately I think I do feel like that, like I definitely feel at risk.

In contrast to Rebecca, who was certain she would test negative, Lori's feelings about her risk are consistent with Finkler's (2001: 244) findings that women with family histories think in terms of 'when I get cancer' rather than 'if I get cancer'. Lori explained her family had not been open about her mother's illness:

> I don't feel like people told me what was going on really and ... even when she had a bone metastases I wasn't told that it was life threatening ... and

it's definitely weird that my family didn't really discuss, when it came time to discuss breast cancer, they didn't actually tell me the real risks and actually the first time my mom had breast cancer they didn't even use the word cancer, they just sort of said a lump in her breast, and it was like a long time before I overheard a nurse saying it ... And so, I do think that's kind of weird.

When I referred to Lori's family as being 'secretive', she did not see it as secrecy but as a reluctance to confront big issues and not knowing how to talk about them:

We never really like ... sat down and had a family meeting or anything like that or talked honestly when my mum had cancer or after her death really ... when it comes to talking about cancer and sorts of issues around genetic mutations, I think we don't communicate that well.

We discussed whether Lori's young age at the time of her mother's cancer may have partly explained her family's reluctance to discuss her mother's illness, as a means to protect her. It is difficult to know whether the family was being secretive or just struggling to come to terms with the loss of Lori's mother. Regardless of the reason, Lori was very clear that her family was not open about her mother's disease and she had to pick up bits and pieces of information through conversations she overheard. She did recall a conversation where her grandmother told her that 'your mother would not forgive herself' if she had passed on a faulty gene to Lori and her sister. This suggests that Lori's mother did feel guilty about possibly being a gene carrier and passing the risk on to her daughters, and this may have been a contributing factor to the reluctance to discuss it with them.

The most striking case of secrecy and silence was that of Susan, Anna and Jennifer's family, and the different responses each of these women had to this secrecy. Susan and Anna had lost their mother to breast cancer when they were in their early and mid-twenties respectively. Anna was the eldest daughter and the first person from the family I interviewed. While Anna had helped to care for her mother throughout her illness, her mother hid it from most people in the family, including her other daughter, Susan. Anna had sought the genetics referral when she was approaching the age at which her mother had become ill, and this had required the investigation of her family history. In the process Anna uncovered many incidences of breast cancer and other cancers that nobody had ever discussed. She started to contact relatives and discovered that most people were unaware of the history of cancer in the family:

I was talking to my cousin [referring to Jennifer] and just sort of tried to see if we all had an awareness of what had been going on in the past in our family, and obviously not ... but still actually even my own immediate circle of family, it's not something we are commonly sharing, and I suppose people just don't actually have a great awareness and it's not something that's that easy to start a conversation about.

Anna described other female relatives who had hidden the details of their breast cancer from their daughters, and a lot of mystery surrounding cancer in general within her extended family. She attributed her mother's reticence to simply not wanting people to make a fuss and start asking a lot of uncomfortable and difficult questions. Anna thought her mother may have inherited this trait of keeping things in:

> My cousin's mother when she died ... her own children were unaware because it wasn't talked about at all outside of one or two people. Nobody really knew, so again that's probably why my mother ... inherited that through her own mother, that sort of reticence to talk about herself so I could understand I would probably be the same, you know. It is very hard ... because it tends to frighten people off, it does. I think it still does.

When I interviewed Anna's sister Susan, the silence surrounding her mother's illness appeared to be more than mere reticence to talk about cancer. It was only near the end of her mother's ten-year battle with breast cancer that Susan was informed of her mother's disease. Susan was still a teenager at the time and tried to get more information from her mother about her illness, but her family was so resistant that they sent her to see a psychotherapist:

> And in fact when ... I said I wanted to get more information out of my mum, she sent me to basically speak to a psychotherapist, to talk my stuff out ... so you know they shoved me out the door 'cuz I wanted to talk about this breast cancer which was like shhhhhh.

Jennifer described the pain of not knowing how sick her much loved aunt was:

> I didn't know, I didn't know until the last few months of her life. I know she'd been diagnosed for eight years and I can't, looking back, I cannot believe how naïve and blind I was, totally blind actually ... I didn't pick up on it. I must have been unbelievably stupid but I didn't pick up until my brother was sent to tell me, that's kind of how things work in this family, and even then I was told that she, aunty, was a private lady and she just didn't want people to know and that was her way and I have to respect that so even then I never actually talked to her. I sent her little cards just you know expressing my feelings but we never, never, it's bizarre, I never said anything, it was almost as though we just had to carry on ... which made me go the other way afterwards because afterwards I was like, I was reading every book I could lay my hands on ... because the *fear of, whispering, and hush hush and secrecy* ... it just makes things really worse actually. [emphasis added]

Jennifer's reaction to the secrecy was to obtain as much information as possible about genetic breast cancer.

I was struck by how deeply the secrecy had been felt by all the members of the extended family. Susan described what had clearly been a very upsetting and traumatic experience for her:

> I was very close with my mum, my father used to describe us as two peas in a pod … so it was very devastating for me when she died … but when she was unwell … and I wanted to talk and try and get more information about the family from her and found that she was a very closed secretive person, and I grew to believe that also was not in her favour, and she wanted to keep her illness to herself which I felt was a big mistake for her … you see when she died the family was in utter shock, 'cuz nobody knew she was unwell.

Following her mother's death, during the traditional Jewish mourning period of seven days known as shivah, the extended family members were so shocked that Susan and her immediate family had spent the entire time trying to comfort them rather than receive consolation and support themselves. Just like Rachel, Susan has an additional non-genetic theory as to why her mother got breast cancer, related to her secretive nature and tendency to keep her feelings in. While Rachel's dissimilar physical appearance to her sister and aunt with breast cancer reassures her, Susan's close physical resemblance to her mother made her extremely concerned that she would develop breast cancer just as her mother did. Being physically or emotionally similar to a relative who had breast cancer made women feel more at risk of getting the disease themselves. One of the first things Susan told me was that she was feeling very anxious because she was approaching the age her mother was when she got ill and was very worried about not being around to see her two young children grow up. Susan had been tested for the BRCA gene mutations but had changed her mind repeatedly about whether she actually wanted the result. She was clearly feeling uncertain about what she would do with the information. By the time I interviewed Susan, her sister Anna had already received her genetic testing results:

> Anna went for her results. *I've forgotten what she said actually* and I postponed mine because … I decided I didn't want to know but now I've decided I do want to know … I think for my children's sake maybe I'll know and then I'll just tuck it away somewhere in my mind, and when they're older you know we'll broach the subject 'cuz *unfortunately you know they will have to know.* [emphasis added]

Similar to the women described earlier, Susan's forgetting her sister's test results had struck me as a way of managing her very high anxiety about getting breast cancer and the implications for her children, which was evident throughout the interview. Susan felt very conflicted about whether she wanted to have the results of her test:

> I was like no, yes, no, yes, no, you know ... I'm still a bit unsure really how it's going to make any difference, um, and will it make me worry more, I don't want it to make me worry more ... So that's my only concern with knowing, will it make me worry, so I might still cancel the appointment ... I'm still having second thoughts ... because on the one hand I think I should know for the kids but like I said ... with me you never know, I could start becoming introspective which is not a good thing.

Susan's anxiety about whether or not she wanted her results had made me feel very concerned because she had already had the genetic test and so it was rather late to be questioning if she wanted to know her status or not. Yet Susan feels a genetic responsibility (Hallowell 1999) to get the information for her children's sake despite the fact that she may not want to know herself. Similar to Rachel, she was also concerned that it could make her worry more and even possibly cause her to get breast cancer. Hallowell (1999) notes that high-risk women were prepared to compromise their own need 'not to know' for the sake of others, and in particular their daughters. Rothenberg (1997) argues that the perceived responsibility women feel to have the test for their children's sake, despite not wanting it themselves, is a form of coercion. Although, as we have seen above, there is also evidence that women may refuse to have the test to avoid certain decisions, possible guilt and responsibility they may feel for passing on the mutations.

Susan's sister Anna did not have children and acknowledged this alleviates some of the potential anxiety of being a carrier:

> If I'm not having children I'm not perpetuating it, but it could be harder for my sister if she knows there's a potential that there's still a risk that her children could pass it on down the line.

Rather than a responsibility to her children, Anna feels a responsibility to her mother:

> I mean I can learn more about me and my past than perhaps was available to my mother. You know if she'd had some information then you know doctors had known then it might have helped but you know that was back in the early 1980s ... as I said just respect the fact that my mother died at an early age from something that perhaps she had no control over but that *I can just live my life as best I can for her*. You know that's still important to me. [emphasis added]

Anna feels a duty to find out as much as she can about her risk out of respect for her mother, while her sister Susan feels a similar obligation for her children. Anna recognizes the implications for future generations, despite not having children herself, while also wanting to have testing for the sake of her mother, as a way of creating something good out of her death. Genetic testing for breast cancer creates a link not only with future generations but also with women from previous generations and acts as a way of memorializing lost mothers and sisters.

Anna had also posed a lot of questions during our interview about the utility of knowing your genetic status and what you were supposed to do with the information:

> Of course if you've got that knowledge, is that good knowledge for everybody automatically? I mean what I am going to do with the information? … I don't know, I haven't really sort of thought it through … what it's going to make me feel because I think, I think I would presumably rather know to be honest.

In Susan's case, she was clearly changing her mind about wanting the test results and did not seem prepared for what would happen following the result. She had asked me a lot of questions about the management options, and when we discussed prophylactic mastectomy, Susan had her own understanding of why this would not reduce her risk. Because her mother's cancer had spread beyond the breast, she did not see how removing the breast tissue would reduce her risk of breast cancer. While I understood Susan's reasoning, her mother's primary cancer was in the breast and prophylactic mastectomy does significantly reduce the risk of developing breast cancer and secondary cancers that may arise from the primary breast cancer. She then explained that she would not want to have a mastectomy because it would raise too many body issues for her anyway. When we discussed the risk of ovarian cancer, this presented even more complications. Her mother had had a hysterectomy at some point and Susan thought this had contributed to her mother developing breast cancer. I did not have any knowledge of why her mother had undergone a hysterectomy; however, removal of the ovaries is one of the options offered to BRCA carriers because it effectively eliminates the risk of ovarian cancer and also significantly reduces the risk of developing breast cancer. But Susan thought removing the ovaries would increase the likelihood of getting breast cancer, not prevent it. On top of this, Susan was ritually observant and did not think Jewish law would permit her to remove her ovaries:

SUSAN: I mean Halachically [referring to Jewish law known as Halacha] I don't think I could remove the ovaries.

JM: Is that true?

SUSAN: I don't know I just read an article recently about it not being Halachic to have your tubes tied unless there was a medical reason, I don't know if this would construe that type of reasoning.

Based on the Jewish rulings related to genetics and screening (described in chapter one), and since removal of the ovaries could be life-saving in Susan's case and she had already had her children, it is likely that most rabbis would rule that it was acceptable for her to have her ovaries removed.

A few days after our interview, Susan emailed me and told me that she had attended her clinic appointment and unfortunately 'it was not good news'. I felt incredibly sympathetic as I understood how upsetting this must have been for her and how unprepared she was for this information. When I discussed the situation with Kathy, her genetic counsellor, she told me the consultation had been very difficult because Anna's test result came back indicating that she was not a carrier but unfortunately Susan's result showed she was a carrier. Susan's appointment had not gone well and apparently she had just shut down and did not want any information from the genetic counsellor. I explained that I had just seen Susan a few days earlier and she was very ambivalent about wanting the results and was going through a difficult and anxious time regarding her mother's death and genetic testing. The genetic counsellor told me that she had had no idea any of that was going on, although Kathy did confide that she sometimes wondered whether the test was offered too easily to Ashkenazi patients. I was so relieved to hear her say this and I shared with her my concerns about this particular family not having had enough information before being offered the test. She agreed with me but said that Ashkenazi patients seem to demand the test and not really want to have a lot of discussion about it or reveal how they felt about it. She told me they asked for genetic testing like 'ordering a burger and fries'. Other clinicians and genetic counsellors I encountered frequently referred to specific characteristics of their Ashkenazi patients, especially that they were particularly demanding. I was reminded of the complexities, difficulties and ambivalence felt by everyone involved in the process of genetic testing for the BRCA mutations, including me, the clinical staff and the families undergoing testing, and of what can happen when assumptions are made about entire groups of people such as Ashkenazi Jews.

Opening up communication

Despite the anxiety about risk and the accompanying silence that I encountered, Susan, Anna and Jennifer's family is an example of how being genetically at risk was creating 'a network of relations' (Novas and Rose 2000) that required opening up communication between distant relatives and undoing the individual and secretive nature of the past as new relationships were being forged between relatives who were previously not in contact with one another. Anna had instigated the search into the family history of cancer by approaching relevant members of the large extended family and trying to gather information about cancer and raise awareness so that women could get on screening programmes. Anna appeared to be taking on the role of raising awareness within the entire network of relatives. This appealed to Jennifer's desire to keep things in the open and she had attempted to organize a special family event for the women to openly discuss the history and risk of genetic breast cancer. She had arranged food and a venue but her efforts were 'completely ambushed' as the women began to ring up and suggest that the men be invited as well and it become a party instead. Jennifer described her family's reaction as follows:

> It just struck me as kind of odd that my attempt just to have a sort of women's group within my own family was kind of viewed as 'oh you mustn't do that' and it got scuppered and it never happened. And I felt quite sad about that, and I kind of thought well I'll have to go elsewhere for women's groups 'cuz it's not gonna happen in my family.

Jennifer had not intended for the family event to be only to discuss breast cancer with the women in her family, but she just wanted to be able to 'air it and discuss it' with them. Despite this failed attempt, it was clear that Anna and Jennifer were changing the family dynamics by getting people to talk about and acknowledge a family history that had been hidden until now.

Conclusion

The previous chapters have demonstrated that genetics can reiterate pre-existing ways in which Ashkenazi Jews conceive of themselves and their history, and this chapter began by showing that genealogy tracing is another practice that reinforces connections with ancestors and familial origins. Family history tracing also plays an integral role in assessing women's genetic risk of breast cancer, and this process can bring family and kin closer to the dead, whom they must recall to account for their genetic heritage, which may promote a sense of continuity with the past, even if it is based on adversity (Finkler 2001: 246). Connerton (1989) describes the ways in which memories can be amassed, conveyed and preserved through the body. He examines the role of bodily practices, ceremony and performance as mechanisms that convey memory through the body. In this chapter, we have seen how family histories of disease and genetic mutations are also ways in which memory can be conveyed. When thinking about their risk of genetic breast cancer, women were inevitably reminded of their mother's, sister's and grandmother's illnesses, and at times of their own breast cancer. These memories were often expressed corporeally, including breasts that were similar to their relatives, surgical scars and having physical and emotional similarities to relatives with breast cancer. Yet these memories were painful and reminded women of the possibility that they too might become ill and leave children or family members behind. Remembering could therefore be accompanied by anxiety, worry and a tendency to forget. Forgetting was complex and appeared to be a strategy for dealing with many of the anxieties and painful memories that were raised by being at increased risk of genetic breast cancer. There were indications that some women, or their mothers, felt guilt about possibly being a mutation carrier and responsibility for passing on genetic mutations that could put their own daughters at risk (the subject of the next chapter). This could lead to a state of denial about the genetic risk or a refusal to undergo testing. Beyond forgetting, there were also stories of a much more explicit silencing of women's family histories of breast cancer, which may have been a result of the history of shame and stigma associated with cancer (Clow 2001, Proctor 1999, Sontag 1990).

That silence and forgetfulness are unique to Ashkenazi Jewish women is not a conclusion that can be drawn from the material; they probably reflect a more generalized way in which families and women deal with many of the difficult issues raised by having a family history of breast cancer. However, the women described in this chapter expressed a significant amount of anxiety and worry, including the possibility of developing cancer in future or having a recurrence, the effectiveness of screening, decisions to undergo prophylactic surgery, whether or not to be genetically tested and guilt about passing mutations to their children. The emotional costs were relatively high, and some women felt pressure to have the test for their children, for their mothers, for Jews in general, or because the knowledge was simply available. Therefore the 'right not to know' may not be realizable for many women (Kenen 1996). In discussing prenatal genetic testing and counselling, Petersen (2003: 193) notes that a decision not to utilize such information is seen increasingly as irresponsible, if not reckless, and as transgressing the rights of the unborn. According to Petersen, the development of a new technology carries the strong expectation that that technology will be applied. Practitioners feel compelled to use the technologies and individuals are expected to want to use them in order to make 'responsible' decisions.

If Ashkenazi Jewish women are more frequently identified in clinical encounters and more frequently offered or referred for genetic counselling or testing than other women, then one unintended consequence is that they may face these difficult and stressful choices more often than other women. This is especially concerning given that mutations are not found in most cases, yet despite this women will still be designated 'high risk' and so forced to face some very difficult decisions about how to manage this risk with the limited management options available. Thus there may be significant, and unintended, emotional consequences for Ashkenazi Jewish women.

This chapter focused on the past and memories; the following chapter turns to the implications of genetic breast cancer for future generations.

6 Future generations

The genetic future – the quality of life that potential offspring will have in terms of genetic illness – now becomes an ethical problem for each risky individual in the genetic present.

(Novas and Rose 2000: 505)

The previous chapter explored how genetic breast cancer provides a link with previous family members and is a way in which memories can be sustained, although family histories also induced painful memories, anxiety and worry that could be forgotten and silenced. This chapter turns to the implications of genetic breast cancer for future generations and the genetic responsibility women experienced for perpetuating genetic breast cancer or mutations. Genetics reveals information not only about individuals but also about biological relationships and kin, and one consequence is that it is inevitably also information about others (Hallowell 1999: 106). As a result, genetic knowledge of disease may induce a sense of genetic responsibility for those who are at risk and reshape obligations and concerns regarding marriage, having children and other aspects of life, such as pursuing a career and organizing financial affairs (Hallowell 1999, Novas and Rose 2000). While the notion of genetic responsibility has received much attention (Hallowell 1999, Hallowell et al. 2006, Lawton et al. 2007, Novas and Rose 2000), less attention has been paid to the role of blame in accounts of genetic responsibility. Arribas-Ayllon et al. (2008a: 1530) use the term 'blame-responsibility' to describe how families and individuals allocate or mitigate blame when dealing with genetic test results which may generate responsibility through self-blame, guilt or 'other-oriented blame'. This chapter focuses on the temporal nature of women's accounts that located responsibility, and allocated blame, for genetic disease in the past, present and future. Once again the collective history of Ashkenazi Jews, this time in terms of marriage and reproductive patterns, is intertwined with the explanation for disease and the implications for future generations. A contradiction may arise between the pre-existing sense of responsibility women feel to reproduce future generations of Jews and the responsibility of producing healthy breast-cancer-free children. This chapter includes interview extracts from non-high-risk individuals, including men, in order to illustrate the importance of endogamy and how the ultra-Orthodox were viewed.

In chapter one we saw that the increased incidence of genetic disease among Ashkenazi Jews is attributed to the processes of genetic drift and the founder effect; that is, a population with a small number of founding members, at least one of whom carries a genetic mutation, increases in size but the population remains closed so the mutation is maintained at higher frequency (Burchard et al. 2003). Ashkenazi Jewish history exemplifies the founder effect and genetic drift as Ashkenazi Jews are descended from a small number of founding ancestors who remained geographically separated in small villages (called shtetls) and were reproductively closed primarily through endogamy (Kahn 2005). Endogamy is the custom of marrying only within the limits of defined communities, tribes or clans (Bittles 2005). Endogamy among Ashkenazi Jews was internally mandated through religious and cultural tenets that endorsed marrying other Jews, and externally imposed through laws that prohibited marriage to non-Jews (Markel 1997). For the Ashkenazi population, one consequence of their history of endogamy is that the frequency of disease-causing alleles did not decrease but remained at increased incidence because when a couple marries it is more likely that both people will be carriers and produce offspring who either carry a single copy of the gene or inherit two copies and exhibit disease.

Another reproductive pattern that can lead to an increased incidence of disease among populations is consanguinity (Bittles 2005). Genetically, consanguinity is defined as marriage between people who are second cousins or closer (Modell and Darr 2002). Endogamy and consanguinity are not the same thing, but endogamous populations may also have a history of consanguinity. Consanguineous marriages did play a significant role in the history and development of the Jewish population, and many early biblical marriages were consanguineous for a number of historical reasons (Goodman 1979). First, Jewish communities were often small and isolated from one another. which restricted the choice of marriage partners. Second, government and religious laws prohibited Jews from marrying non-Jews. Third, Jews often chose to marry within families because of socio-economic or religious ties and prearrange these marriages from a young age. Consanguineous marriages can strengthen family ties, allow men and women to find partners with relative ease, protect the woman's status and lead to better and more stable relationships between in-laws (Modell and Darr 2002). Finally, some forms of marriage between family members are sanctioned by Jewish law, known as Halacha (Goodman 1979).

Consanguinity is most commonly found in North Africa, the Middle East and Central and South Asia and is relatively uncommon in Europe, North America and Australasia (Bittles 2005, Modell and Darr 2002). In Western societies, consanguinity is generally viewed as causing physical and mental incapacity and is referred to as 'inbreeding' and viewed with prejudice (Modell and Darr 2002). Historically, the ill health of the Jews was frequently associated with their sexual practices, primarily the tendency to marry young or to marry blood relatives (Gilman 1985). Inbreeding was associated with morally corrupt and incestuous sexually deviant practices that further stigmatized Jews and contributed to the sense of Jew as other, and represented confusion between endogamous marriage and incestuous inbreeding which are not synonymous. According to Gilman (1985), the idea that Jews are inbred is an inaccurate representation of the Jews and a tool that has been used to keep them separate, while at the same time Jews themselves held these views. Goodman and Goodman (1982) contend that Eastern European Jews were unaware they were undergoing consanguineous marriages because they were frequently dispersed due to persecution and then re-encountered one another and unsuspectingly married a distant cousin who shared a common ancestor with a genetic mutation. While this practice has been rapidly declining, prearranged, and sometimes consanguineous, marriages still take place among ultra-Orthodox Jews (Goodman 1979: 463, Levene 2005).

Recollecting Jewish reproductive history

This section describes how individuals temporally located genetic responsibility for the increased risk of disease among Ashkenazi Jews in their collective endogamous reproductive past. The topic of the endogamous history of Ashkenazi Jews arose in every interview and there was widespread acceptance of these practices. The most common way individuals described Jewish reproductive history was in terms of 'cousin marriage'.

When Elizabeth and I discussed why the risk of genetic breast cancer was increased for Ashkenazi Jews, she explained it as follows:

> I kept thinking about why, and why has it been ... but I've always honestly wrote it off as something for example, many illnesses in royal circles 'cuz they tended to intermarry. This is what could have happened within the Jewish community as well ... so we are sort of descendants and sometimes they had to marry cousins and things like that so the probability of something has been increased in intermarrying within the family so, um, trying to think whether there are other groups of people that would be sort of in a similar way be *more in danger* by something like that, I can't think of anything. [emphasis added]

Elizabeth acknowledges the 'dangers' of being descendants of cousins who married one another, while at the same time she likens marriage between relatives to the situation in royal families. She was not alone in making such comparisons; according to Sarah:

> I say look guys, my relatives were all first cousins, because nobody wasn't their cousin you know ... you look at the Royal Family, I mean I know everybody says that ... but they've all married their cousins for years ... yeah and they talked about it with Princess Di, didn't they? That she was

like a good brood mare, you know, good breeding stock, to kind of improve the strain, yeah.

Sarah had two much loved dogs who wandered in and out throughout the interview. She pointed out the health implications for dog breeding:

I've been reading about this one guy who was a fanatic lurcher breeder and ... he had to keep bringing in outcrosses to keep his strain healthy ... they were just obviously breeding very closely related dogs and they were getting all sorts of strange weaknesses, so it's such an interesting subject, isn't it?

Both Elizabeth and Sarah acknowledge the 'dangers' and 'weaknesses' that can arise from breeding too closely, yet they simultaneously naturalize these practices through their references to the Royal Family and animal husbandry. Sarah's comment 'that nobody wasn't their cousin' and Elizabeth's that sometimes 'they had to' marry cousins express the impossibility of finding a marriage partner who was not related, which refers to both the historical living conditions of Ashkenazi Jews in shtetls and discrimination that prohibited marriage to non-Jews.

Mira was in her early sixties and had developed breast cancer at the age of 49. It had been discovered at an early stage and she had been treated successfully. She had not undergone genetic testing. I interviewed Mira in her home one afternoon and we spent many hours talking about genetic breast cancer and Jewish identity. After I turned the tape off, we went into the kitchen and Mira introduced me to her husband and mentioned the topic of our discussion. He told me that their parents' generation had all 'married their cousins' because they lived in small communities and there were not enough people who were not relatives to marry. Mira agreed and they spoke of this in a very matter of fact way as an accepted part of their background. I was reminded of my own family and how my mother frequently used to refer to the fact that her Eastern European grandparents, my great-grandparents, were all married to their cousins. I do not know if this was actually true of my great-grandparents or was more a sort of myth about Jewish historical marriage practices.

When Laura and I discussed the increased risk of genetic breast cancer, she said:

Well the Jewish breeding from a smaller um mass of people who are related ... not intermarriage but within a very small sample or you know a very distinct line. You're gonna double the risk of anything like Tay-Sachs, aren't you? I mean like Greek people with thalassemia and sickle cell disease for Caribbean Africans, so you know you're gonna do that, you're gonna double the risk aren't you? Um, it's like these four kittens [referring to her own kittens] you know if they had kittens with the brother next door the only defects they've got are gonna be doubled. I mean I'm not a scientist.

Laura's comparisons to other groups with disease, such as Greeks and Africans, are used to point out that Jews are not unique in their increased risk. Like Sarah, she uses her own pets and references to animal breeding both to naturalize and to describe the potential 'defects' that can arise from close breeding. Laura had direct experience of first cousins marrying on both her mother's and her father's side of the family, including her own generation of relatives. She described the children of these marriages:

> Their little boys are fantastic just as the girls of the first cousins were fantastic ... And on my father's side the children are extremely intelligent, absolutely ugly [laughter] ... So do I think interbreeding is a bad thing? Well I think if you go to the Blue Ridge Mountains of Virginia and see the hillbillies you probably would think it was a bad thing but how can you condemn people for doing it? ... I think it was very common when they were all in Russia, and environs, and I think it's probably a natural thing. I mean when you look at farmers, where do they breed their animals? I mean there's inter-sibling production there isn't there?

Laura's description of cousin marriage and inbreeding is ambivalent and expresses contrasting views. On the one hand, it is a 'natural thing' that one cannot 'condemn' people for doing and which regularly occurs in farm breeding. Yet, on the other hand, the children of cousin marriage in her own family have been affected in terms of their physical appearance, and Laura's use of the derogatory term 'hillbillies' also implies there are negative and morally problematic consequences of inbreeding, but only in certain contexts (such as the Blue Ridge Mountains).

Anna also related the increased risk to historical reproductive patterns:

> But it's interesting to understand this background because ... presumably it's all through intermarriage. It's sort of fascinating ... well it must be cousins, I presume it's coming through cousins, I suppose we have no idea of what background, I mean what sort of communities they lived in and one assumes it was an acceptable way of life in being introduced to what must be your first or your second cousin.

Anna mitigates moral judgement on these 'communities' by saying that she assumes this must have been 'an acceptable way of life'. Yet she simultaneously places these practices firmly in the past, a temporal strategy that distances Anna from, and allocates responsibility to, history.

On a few occasions, individuals would ask me to explain why there was an increased risk of genetic disease among Ashkenazi Jews. I tried to delay as long as possible before explaining the reasons as I wanted to uncover individuals' own understanding about why these genetic mutations might arise. Very early on in my interview with Jennifer, she told me that she did not understand why these genetic mutations were more common in Ashkenazi

Jews and that she was hoping it was something I could help her to understand.

JM: So can I ask you what you know about the connection with being Ashkenazi?

JENNIFER: Well all I know and I don't understand why it is, all I know is that Ashkenazi Jewish women have a higher chance of getting breast cancer. I don't quite know why, I don't know if it's the same for Sephardi women, I don't know if it's related to diet, um, if it is we all grew up with the same diet pretty much um, what do you know? Can you help? Can you tell me?

Jennifer had thought the risk of genetic breast cancer might be related to the Jewish diet and we had then discussed the founder mutations. She was aware of the history of close marriages and even though she had not directly connected it to the increased risk of disease, she said:

> I know the history, you know, was that we were in tiny shtetls so I guess it makes sense, um and it's just one of those things … we've all seen *Fiddler on the Roof*, so I guess you know it does make sense, they don't marry that far out really do they? It's different today I suppose there's a lot more, well for a start we're not living in tiny little shtetls. We live in big cities and we're just sort of out there much more, and everything has changed beyond measure what our great grandparents would have imagined um, so I suppose it's probably reducing as well now, maybe … even if you were still marrying a Jewish person, it wouldn't necessarily be from your village, it could be from Birmingham or you know whatever so that the kind of risk that kind of intermarriage is probably reducing now.

Similar to the other women described, Jennifer associates cousin marriage with the way of life in Eastern European shtetls, but she explicitly distances these practices from those of today.

Women temporally displaced and mitigated genetic responsibility for disease to the endogamous history of Ashkenazi Jews, thereby creating distance between themselves and these practices. The following section turns to a discussion of where blame and responsibility were allocated in the present.

The ultra-Orthodox as 'other'

The ultra-Orthodox are the most theologically conservative branch of Judaism. They are made up of different sects and do not form a single unified community, although they do have some common characteristics (Dein 2002, Raz 2010). They live in isolated communities, strictly adhere to Jewish religious law, limit their contact with the secular world, undergo arranged marriages and have a high birth rate (Prainsack 2007, Raz 2010). The ultra-Orthodox movement arose in eighteenth-century Europe as a direct response to the many Jews who were promoting a more reformed type of Judaism that would allow them to assimilate and become part of life outside the ghettos. These Jews went on to form the more liberal branches of Judaism such as the Modern Orthodox (also known as Conservative in the US and Canada), Liberal and Reform movements. The ultra-Orthodox continue to adhere as closely as possible to the way of life of their Eastern European ancestors in previous generations, and for some of the individuals interviewed they symbolized the continuation of historical practices of the Jews in the present day.

No ultra-Orthodox individuals were interviewed for this study, and the primary reason was that very few were referred to the clinics attended during the research, something the genetic counsellors attributed to their use of private health care rather than the National Health Service. Therefore, the purpose of this section is not to make claims about the ultra-Orthodox but rather to illustrate the ways in which less religious individuals conceptualized the ultra-Orthodox in contrast to themselves.

Michelle was a ritually observant Jewish woman who lived in a London neighbourhood with a large Jewish population that included many ultra-Orthodox Jews. In describing her neighbourhood, she said:

> So you've got a lot of young frum [Yiddish word for devout] people moving in, you know in their early twenties covering their hair already, and you know they're very very frum, which is wonderful I think. Sometimes it feels a bit like a ghetto, you know, which I don't always think is such a good thing ... because I think if you take people like us ... you know they're not necessarily always gonna mix with Jewish people whereas the frum community will only ever mix with their own whereas we won't.

For Michelle, the large number of ultra-Orthodox Jews in her neighbourhood is a positive sign that the Jewish community is still thriving and growing, while their presence is also reminiscent of Eastern European ghettos. While Michelle embraces them, she simultaneously distances herself from them by referring to 'people like us' as opposed to the 'frum'. The ultra-Orthodox were seen as being closed to outsiders and this separated them from not only non-Jews but also other less religious Jews as well:

> I think what worries me is um when you know when you see for example the very Orthodox who have all these children, and many of them have special needs. And it's I mean obviously it's sometimes the woman's age, but also you don't know because you don't know where somewhere along the line there may be an interfamily relation that's caused the problem. And I think that's very sad.

Michelle's daughter had been born with a genetic disease called oculocutaneous albinism, which is not specifically at increased incidence among Ashkenazi Jews although she had attended a support group for Jewish mothers of children with special needs. Her attendance at this group had exposed her to ultra-Orthodox women whom she did not usually socialize with; in describing the group, she said:[1]

> Probably 70 per cent were like me and 30 per cent were very frum, cover their hair and had lots of children, and you know there was one woman and she had five children … and she was like in her late forties when she had her daughter and this kid had special needs … And there was another girl there oh my god, she must have been at least 10 years younger than me … I think she had seven and was pregnant with her eighth … and her twins, which were her sixth and seventh, had special needs, well I'm not bloody surprised! Because somewhere along the line, you're gonna have a kid that's not gonna be right and I think that's more worrying … these are kids that have got major, major problems, and that I think is dreadful … and that's obviously genetic, somewhere along the lines something has happened.

Michelle 'worries' about the marriage and reproductive practices of the ultra-Orthodox, including a high birth rate, late births and the possibility of 'interfamily relations', and associates these practices with their ill health. Mira lived in the same area of North London as Michelle. She distinguished the ultra-Orthodox as completely separate from her and repeated many times throughout our interview how the high birth rate was very unhealthy for the women and children, referring to the women as 'baby machines'.

Michael was a young ritually observant British man who did not have a family history of disease, but when I asked him about his understanding of genetic disease among Ashkenazi Jews, he said:

> I guess because of the history of Jews marrying Jews the genes got into the system and stayed there for I don't know hundreds of years or something but … I don't really think about it, it's not anything that really affects me and I don't think ever will, not really. The only thing I am aware of is in the very ultra-Orthodox community they all kind of marry their cousins and then things go very wrong there, which I'm not intending on doing. So that is the only thing I suppose about genetic diseases that I am aware of really.

Michael places close marriages firmly in the past, while at the same time 'cousin marriage' is a current practice specific to the ultra-Orthodox. However, he does not associate himself in any way with them and therefore does not worry about his own future health or risk of disease.

Individuals cast the ultra-Orthodox as 'other' (Michael and Birke 1994) to create distance between themselves and what they saw as the unhealthy practices being perpetuated by the ultra-Orthodox. According to Michael and Birke (1994), by contrasting themselves with various 'others', individuals can present their own behaviour in a positive, moral or superior light, while simultaneously distancing themselves from potential stigma, shame or immorality. The use of 'others' can be relative so that some groups are only cast as 'other' in specific contexts. In contrast to the majority of individuals who were disassociating themselves from the ultra-Orthodox, Rachel questioned her genetic proximity to them. She described the ultra-Orthodox in her neighbourhood:

> I mean that's just totally alien, but it's probably totally alien to most people 'cuz it's so extreme and closed. I mean but if that's the same gene pool that's carrying this gene [referring to BRCA]. That would be the same gene pool, those are Ashkenazi Jews then aren't they?

Rachel was questioning this categorization of 'other' because, despite her efforts to separate herself from the 'alien' ultra-Orthodox, the BRCA genes actually reinforced the interrelatedness of all Ashkenazi Jews.

These reproductive practices were also seen to have direct consequences for increasing the number of BRCA mutation carriers in future generations, and according to Laura:

> Amazing this resurgence of the very Orthodox and how they're having bigger families ... if one of them, you know, if the mother's got BRCA1 BRCA2 it could be the whole family and ... one generation is 10, the next generation could be 30 ... with the Orthodox they're coming back, they'll have 10 kids each and that multiplies the risk for them too, and the boys as well.

For Laura, the 'resurgence' of the ultra-Orthodox, and their large families, are both amazing and potentially blameworthy for perpetuating the number of BRCA mutation carriers.

Although Anna avoids directly naming them and instead refers to 'some parts of the community', she also questioned the role of the ultra-Orthodox in increasing the BRCA mutations:

> I mean it's becoming very watered down but it is still there you know. Is it a risk people continuing to have children and perpetuating it, albeit tiny? You know will it just eradicate itself eventually or is it being perpetuated in some parts of the community more than others? ... So there may well be these same practices of close marriages, which is continuing to perpetuate the uh existence of more cancers, but ... would it make people stop is an interesting question.

Anna wonders if knowing close marriages were perpetuating disease might lead individuals to stop, and the following section turns to the final temporal account of responsibility and blame, that of reproductive consequences and future generations.

Marrying in: implications for future generations

Endogamy remains important to many Jews who currently feel a responsibility, as well as familial pressure, to marry other Jews in order to preserve Judaism and ensure the survival of future generations. This is related to political and cultural concerns that once someone marries a non-Jew, they will not provide their children with a Jewish upbringing and education, an especially important consideration in the current climate of assimilation and decreasing numbers. The number of intermarriages – of Jews marrying non-Jews – has been significantly increasing over the last 40 years and is estimated to be 40–45 per cent in the UK currently (Graham 2004). For some, maintaining the Jewish population is directly associated with the survival of the state of Israel, where political and violent conflict with surrounding Arab states and a decreasing population put the entire Israeli collective body in danger of 'annihilation' (Prainsack and Firestine 2006: 40). In addition, traditional Orthodox Jewish law stipulates that a child must be born to a Jewish mother in order to be considered Jewish. While many liberal and reform branches of Judaism do not adhere to this, being born to a Jewish mother is still seen by many as a necessity to be considered Jewish (as was demonstrated in chapter four).

According to Berman (2010: 94), Jewish intermarriage is a post-war communal obsession, and debates in the last half century reveal a politics of blame and particularly blame of parents. Historically, endogamy was an extremely important mechanism for communal separation. However, in the early twentieth century American Jews began to become increasingly assimilated into American society and tensions arose between 'being American' and religious and ethnic ideals. In the first half of the twentieth century most Jews continued to marry other Jews, so intermarriage was not a particularly salient issue, especially as there were ongoing and persistent concerns about immigrants contaminating and weakening the nation during this period. Social science research at this time endorsed endogamy, as 'interfaith marriages' were found to have higher divorce rates and supposedly negative consequences for the children's identity and development (Berman 2010). In the post-war period, liberal and permissive parenting was highly valued by Jews, yet it was this very permissiveness that was seen to be causing their children's lack of interest in Judaism and endogamy, and contributing to children's belief that they could marry for love. From the 1960s onwards, the increase in Jewish institutions, schools, university programmes, summer camps and organized trips to Israel served to rectify 'inadequate Jewish parenting' and alleviate communal anxiety about intermarriage (Berman 2010: 104). It is within this same context that distinctive 'Jewish diseases' such as Tay-Sachs became powerful common reference points and forms of 'symbolic ethnic identity' (as described in chapter one; see also Wailoo and Pemberton 2006).

The London Jewish Cultural Centre offered a four-week course devoted to this topic called 'Intermarriage – Was It Ever a Good Thing?'. The course allowed attendees to:

> Explore high profile intermarriages in the Bible and other parts of Jewish
> history and consider whether the current concern about intermarriage is a
> new obsession, an ancient approach or just an example of Jews missing the
> point of what's good for them.
>
> (London Jewish Cultural Centre 2007)

The course was attended by a small but varied group of individuals ranging
from 20 to 80 years of age. On the first day all attendees were asked to tell the
group why they were taking the course and most individuals described personal
experiences or concerns regarding intermarriage. One man was the child of
intermarriage, while others were concerned about their own children's intermarriages. One woman indicated that she was just curious about the ways in
which Judaism, and other religions, were 'never really pure' because there were
always outsiders who entered a group. Each week we explored biblical marriages
or stories that involved the marriage of Jews to non-Jews. The course lecturer
repeatedly reminded us that it is anachronistic to project our current understanding of Jewish belonging onto biblical times. There were frequent marriages
between Jews and non-Jews, and if we consider Abraham to be the first Jew,
there would have been no other Jews around for him or his descendants to marry.

The topic of intermarriage and of Jews marrying other Jews arose in every
interview. While not everyone believed it was imperative, 10 (of 19) individuals
felt it was important and had concerns about increasing rates of intermarriage.
Often people wanted to know whether I had a Jewish partner and, at times,
the fact that I did not was a source of common ground and connection,
especially if they themselves or their children also did not. On other occasions
I deliberately did not mention that my partner was not Jewish because individuals had indicated to me how vital they thought it was to have a Jewish
partner and so I felt uncomfortable talking about my personal situation as a
result. Ben was very concerned about the consequences of intermarriage:

> The numbers are dwindling as we speak. Assimilation rates are like
> 50 per cent and I think that's really problematic. I mean we are gonna
> reach a stage at which there are so few Jews in the Diaspora, which is already
> the case, but even fewer ... And also you know, we are so vulnerable now
> because Israel is so vulnerable ... That's a very tenuous situation.

For Ben, maintaining the Jewish population is directly associated with the
survival of the state of Israel. Maintaining a Jewish population that is higher
than the non-Jewish population in Israel is crucial to justifying the continued
existence of a separate Jewish state (Prainsack and Firestine 2006).

For Mira, it was essential that her children marry Jews, but especially her
son because of the requirement to have a Jewish mother:

> I mean my son has always said ... that he would never marry out ... but
> for my daughter her children would still be Jewish and she would bring

them up to be Jewish. But for my son, his children wouldn't be Jewish. You know I think it's a shame that we lose, break the links in the chain.

Marrying out would break the continuity between generations, the 'links in the chain', that Mira sees as critical to being Jewish. While Mira highlights the importance of being born to a Jewish mother, she also implies that, unlike her daughter, her son may not provide his children with a Jewish upbringing if he married someone non-Jewish.

Michelle said that she would be 'devastated' if her children married out, but her reasoning is more explicitly related to passing on a Jewish upbringing:

> But I feel that if I show my children, and I steer them in the right direction then you know they hopefully will keep within their religion and you know, carry it on and on and on. If I don't show them, they can't show their children.

For Elana, who was ritually observant, assimilation represents the downfall of Jews, which she related to biblical history and God's wishes:

> The assimilation, that will be our downfall ... the younger Jewish people, many of them ... are assimilating ... And ask the questions and look at our history and you can see where we've gone down. I mean why did we have to wander for 40 years, why? Because it was to knock out that assimilation from people, and the next generation and the next one after that were as hashem [Hebrew word for God] wanted them to be, but we've gone backwards now.

Daniel described a story to me about a serious non-Jewish girlfriend he had for four years while at university. His parents were so upset by this that they would not allow her into their home.[2] On one occasion they drove for two hours to get to his parents' house and his girlfriend was not allowed 'over the doorstep', so she eventually converted to Judaism. The relationship had broken down in the end but it remained very important to Daniel that he married someone Jewish:

> It's amazing how strong it is – the deep deep desire that the girlfriend should be Jewish, and not just Jewish, but Jewish like me.

Daniel explained that his desire to have a Jewish girlfriend had 'driven him out of certain relationships, breaking my heart in the process, driven me into other ones and I shouldn't have done'. When describing his wish to find a Jewish wife, or 'maiden' as he referred to her, he said:

> I'm not really religiously minded or biblically minded but it conjured up you know Ruths, and Esthers and Miriams and Sarahs, and that idea that

I might draw on that sort of depth of not just rootedness but even a metaphysical rootedness.

Nancy described how significant it had been to her parents that she marry someone Jewish, even though her upbringing was not religious and her parents were 'kind of atheist'. Nancy and her three sisters were encouraged to have Jewish friends and marry Jewish men, which they all did. She had two teenage sons and although she was unsure if it would matter if they married out, she noted 'I might think differently in a few years' time. I mean I might feel that they have a better chance of a successful marriage if they *stay within*' [emphasis added]. For Nancy, endogamy is a way of ensuring a 'successful' marriage through a shared cultural background.

The way in which endogamy reproduces both 'biological' connection (through the need to be born to a Jewish mother, for example) and also 'social' connection (through a Jewish education and upbringing) demonstrates that relatedness was never one thing, and definitively never a matter of either social or biological connection alone (Edwards and Strathern 2000: 154). Reproducing Jews is a result of 'social' and 'biological' processes which can often be conflated (see Kahn 2000) and, just as we saw in chapter four, Jewish identity is itself also a combination and conflation of 'biological' and 'social' domains.

For those women who felt a responsibility to ensure the survival of future generations and maintain Jewish culture through endogamy, there was no apparent conflict between this religious/cultural imperative and the risk of perpetuating genetic disease as a result. Importantly, as will be demonstrated in the following section, this was not always the case.

Marrying out: a dangerous gene pool

According to Goodman (1979), few people would endorse marrying non-Jews as an acceptable means of reducing the rate of genetic disease among Jews. However, for some women with direct experience of genetic disease in the family, marrying out was viewed as a way to reduce the likelihood of future disease. This was connected to women's personal upsetting experiences of breast cancer or caring for ill mothers or sisters with the disease, and their understanding that this illness was the result of the endogamous history of the Jews. Sarah and I discussed her husband:

> He's not Jewish ... there was so much pressure all through my life to marry a nice Jewish boy and you know I think three of us didn't [referring to her sisters], and I think thank God for that, you know nobody ever talks about you know get out there and marry the goyim [Yiddish word for Gentile] because your gene pool needs help [laughter] ... and I *blame it on Jews now*. I mean I just think Jews intermarrying [referring to Jews marrying other Jews] fills me with horror now. [emphasis added]

Sarah's description of the amount of pressure she felt growing up reflects the amount of cultural pressure that is placed on many young Jews to marry someone who is Jewish (as illustrated in the previous section). However, Sarah feels extremely grateful that she did not succumb to this demand, which literally fills her with 'horror' and is directly responsible for creating a gene pool that 'needs help'. Sarah views her own family as being riddled with cancer caused by a genetic mutation resulting from a history of cousin marriage. She also associates ill health in general with Ashkenazi Jews and uses this to explain a different disease suffered by her sister's son:

> And my youngest sister, the one who died [of breast cancer], who also married an Ashkenazi Jew, um ... her younger son had a very odd heart problem, which they also think may have been genetic ... well they don't know but *I blame it on Jews now.* [emphasis added]

This 'other-oriented blame' (Arribas-Ayllon et al. 2008a: 1523) displaces individual responsibility for passing on mutations onto the entire community of Jews (see also Gilman 2003). While others have shown that individuals may feel anger towards or place blame on relatives for the transmission of genetic disease and mutations (Arribas-Ayllon et al. 2008a, 2008b, Hallowell et al. 2006, Lawton et al. 2007), in this context the net of blame is cast more widely to implicate Ashkenazi Jews rather than family members. A genetic counsellor anecdotally reported having an Ashkenazi Jewish patient who was a BRCA mutation carrier and felt very angry with Jews, whom she blamed for the mutations. Unfortunately this woman could not be interviewed as a recent mammogram had revealed a breast lump and she was too anxious to take part in the research.

Sarah believed her marriage to someone who was not Jewish reduced the risk of her passing on a BRCA mutation, which was especially important as she had a daughter:

> And I was sort of reassured at the idea that ... my daughter's 10 and ... I don't worry about my daughter all that much because she is very much like my husband's family in every way ... I mean it doesn't mean she doesn't have the gene, but I doubt she has it on both sides. My husband's nice English Church of England you know so he's not gonna have an Ashkenazi.

Despite the fact that BRCA mutation testing had not revealed a mutation in Sarah's family, she said: 'Well, to me it's obvious that both my parents are carriers [referring to BRCA genes].' Sarah's belief that the BRCA mutations could be inherited from 'both sides' or that both of her parents were carriers indicates that she does not distinguish between dominant and recessive transmission patterns. Unlike recessive diseases, which only manifest when mutations are inherited from both parents, carrying a single copy of a BRCA mutation can cause disease. BRCA mutations cannot be inherited from 'both sides' as a foetus would not survive in utero if it inherited two copies of the same BRCA mutation (a concept known as double lethality). If Sarah is a BRCA mutation carrier, her daughter's risk of inheriting a mutation from her is 50 per cent regardless of her husband's genetic status. However, Sarah sees her husband as healthier simply because he is not Jewish and her daughter's similarity to him and his 'Church of England' family bestows health. Her husband's non-Jewish genes provide an element of protection and for Sarah the solution was clear (emphasis added): 'Marrying out. It doesn't bother me. You know as someone with breast cancer ... it's a *dangerous gene pool.*'

Sarah explicitly associates her feelings about marrying out with her own family history and experience of breast cancer. At the same time, she acknowledges that her views could be problematic because they go against very fundamental religious and cultural tenets within Judaism about the importance of endogamy and producing Jewish offspring:

> Well it's not the kind of thing that they're [Jews] gonna advertise is it? I mean, it goes against absolutely everything ... but then how do you educate people? You don't exactly do it through the synagogue do you – 'whatever you do don't marry another Ashkenazi Jew'?

Helen was a British woman in her mid-seventies. She was retired and lived with her husband. She had breast cancer at 59 and 72 and had undergone genetic testing, but no BRCA mutation was found. Helen expressed equally strong feelings about the need to marry out to prevent further genetic disease, although this was not directly related to her history of breast cancer. Helen's daughter Lily had Bloom syndrome, a rare and incurable recessive genetic disease that occurs with increased incidence among Ashkenazi Jews. She described an incredibly difficult life caring for a severely disabled child, especially when Lily was young. Helen admitted that perhaps if she had not had a daughter with genetic disease, she might feel differently about the importance of marrying someone Jewish, but the reality was that having a disabled child had seriously affected her life. She kept reiterating how much she loved her daughter and I understood that it was important to her that I did not interpret her views as signifying regret over her daughter's birth. Helen had another unaffected daughter who had been determined not to marry someone Jewish because of the risk of having a child with genetic disease, and this had been a contributing factor to her daughter's cancelled engagement to a Jewish man. Helen's unaffected daughter was a carrier of the recessive Bloom syndrome mutation and the man she was engaged to was a carrier of a different recessive disease (Helen could not remember which one). There was no genetic risk of their children being affected with either of these diseases as they are both recessive, but Helen's story suggests that their decision not to marry was a result of the significant emotional impact and distress caused by having a family history of disease rather than a biogenetic understanding of recessive transmission. Helen described how her daughter had married a six-foot tall Australian non-Jewish man and gone on to have two healthy, strong and intelligent children. Similar to Sarah, Helen associated marrying a non-Jewish man with health, strength and good genes that produced healthy offspring.

Joan was a British woman in her sixties who attended a talk I gave at a Reform synagogue in north London. When I mentioned Tay-Sachs, Joan immediately called out loudly to the group: 'Marry out!' Afterwards, Joan approached me and told me about her own family history. She was from a very large ultra-Orthodox family in the United States, although she was no longer ritually observant. She had 76 cousins, indicating the very high birth rate among her relatives. Within her family there was a recessive genetic disease that occurred more often in Ashkenazi Jews, and although she could not remember the name of it, she described it as an awful, frightening and fatal disease. The siblings of two of the individuals who had died of this disease had chosen to marry non-Jews, and she was certain this was to avoid having children with the illness despite the fact that they refused to openly acknowledge this. Joan saw marrying out as an important way to reduce the risk of genetic disease among Ashkenazi Jews.

While Helen and Sarah were the only two high-risk women who endorsed marrying non-Jews, there were other women with family histories of breast cancer who felt that it was still essential for Jews to marry other Jews but that it would be preferable to marry a non-Ashkenazi Jew. Most suggested marrying a Sephardi Jew. Sephardi Jews left the Middle East following the destruction of the second temple (in approximately 70 CE) and settled primarily in Spain as opposed to Eastern Europe. Susan was ritually observant and considered it vital that Jews marry other Jews to maintain the 'people'. Despite this, her strong family history of cancer led her to feel it was important to marry a non-Ashkenazi Jew:

SUSAN: I just hadn't been aware, neither had Anna [her sister], until the end of last year really how much cancer had infiltrated the family but it does seem to be um, diluting, which is normal, um and I can only hope for my kids that it's completely diluted you know. But I will definitely try and steer them in the direction of marrying Sephardis.

JM: Really?

SUSAN: Yes ... because the disposition is generally more for Ashkenazi Jews, and ... I'd try and steer them in the right direction! It's unrealistic but I wouldn't try and discourage them ... because I really don't want them to have to deal with this.

Susan believed the breast cancer genes were being 'diluted' because she did not see as many incidents of breast cancer in her generation, and because some of her relatives had married out. Susan explained that when she was searching for a partner, she had tried to date Sephardi men but it 'just didn't work out' and in the end she had married an Ashkenazi Jewish man. Susan felt that marrying out would provide her children with the best possible future chances of remaining healthy and cancer free, thereby helping them to avoid the significant anxiety that she was facing herself about the possibility of being a carrier and developing breast cancer. After our interview, Susan's genetic test revealed that she was a BRCA mutation carrier and unfortunately her own children's risk of inheriting the mutation remains 50 per cent, regardless of their choice of marriage partner. While marrying out could potentially reduce the overall population risk of BRCA mutations over time, for those women who are carriers, their own children's risk unfortunately cannot be reduced this way because the genes are transmitted in an autosomal dominant fashion. In contrast, population screening and carrier testing for recessive diseases such as Tay-Sachs can have surprising, and perhaps counterintuitive, effects. By allowing Jewish carrier couples to marry and reproduce but avoid having an affected offspring through prenatal screening and abortion of affected foetuses (or pre-implantation genetic diagnosis), the number of children who are born carriers of a single recessive Tay-Sachs allele has actually increased rather than decreased (Motulsky and Fraser 1980). The overall effect is negligible in terms of public health, but noteworthy nonetheless when considering the potential impacts of population screening and genetic testing.

Susan and I continued to talk after I had turned the tape off. She then told me about a serious relationship she had had many years earlier with a man she intended to marry. In the end they broke up, and while there were many reasons for the break up, one contributing factor was his family's concern regarding her mother's breast cancer. Recently she had discovered that this ex-boyfriend's mother had also died of breast cancer, which made her question whether perhaps his family also had a history of breast cancer and believed the marriage could be unhealthy for any future children. Susan is suggesting that her ex-boyfriend's family had carried out their own self-screening programme, as opposed to the formal screening programmes such as those for Tay-Sachs, by making a conscious decision not to encourage a marriage between families who both had a history of the same disease.

Conclusion

The chapter began with accounts of genetic responsibility for breast cancer that were located in the past, and specifically how women associated their risk of genetic disease with a history of endogamy among Ashkenazi Jews, most commonly expressed as 'cousin marriage'. Women's familiarity with this reproductive history is another way in which genetic disease and mutations reiterate pre-existing narratives, in this case a narrative about a shared history of 'cousin marriage'. Women acknowledged the possible negative consequences for genetic disease and ill health, and at times made critical or derogatory references to these reproductive practices (for example referring to 'hillbillies' and 'dangers'). While there was no expression of overt shame about this history, individuals did have various discursive strategies for mitigating any potential responsibility. First, they created temporal distance by placing these practices firmly in the past as something that had happened in Eastern European shtetls. They also naturalized these practices by referring to the frequent use of inbreeding in animal husbandry and farming. By making comparisons with other groups such as the Royal Family, Africans and sickle cell disease, and Mediterranean populations and thalassemia, individuals were pointing out that Jews were not unique in their increased risk of disease or their reproductive history but resembled other populations. These 'moral images' (Agar 2004) helped to mitigate blame and potentially morally problematic aspects of inbreeding because genetic disease occurred in these other groups as well. The moral image of an unfamiliar practice is another more familiar practice chosen for both its similarity to the problematic practice and the fact that it elicits moral reactions of which we are confident (Agar 2004: 39). When individuals referred to Ashkenazi Jewish historical reproductive practices, they used moral images in the form of the Royal Family, Africans and sickle cell disease, thalassemia among Mediterranean populations and even animal breeding to reiterate the fact that these practices were not morally problematic as they happened in other populations as well. Rather than distancing, this was a way of creating proximity and minimizing any difference specific to Jews. Lastly, women also mitigated responsibility by acknowledging that these reproductive practices may not have been the result of choice as discrimination prohibited Jews from marrying non-Jews or confined them to ghettos.

In the present, women allocated blame, and thereby displaced responsibility, to a particular community of Ashkenazi Jews, namely the ultra-Orthodox, and in so doing they contrasted themselves with those they deemed as currently perpetuating problematic behaviour (Arribas-Ayllon et al. 2008a). Arribas-Ayllon et al.'s (2008a: 1522) research on parental decisions to genetically test their children found that accounts of blame reveal strategies for presenting the self as responsible and praiseworthy, either by contrasting the self with those who are irresponsible or by foregrounding aspects of responsible conduct. By contrasting themselves with the ultra-Orthodox, and their high birth rate and perceived tendency to enter into consanguineous marriages, women distanced themselves from genetic responsibility in the present. This did not necessarily prevent women from also embracing certain aspects of the ultra-Orthodox, particularly as symbols of a growing or thriving group of Ashkenazi Jews.

As regards the future, genetic disease undoubtedly brings 'potential futures into the present' and creates concerns and responsibility for future generations (Rose 2007: 18). However, Ashkenazi Jews already feel a responsibility to ensure the survival of future generations of Jews, with endogamy being an important means to achieve this. Yet, it is this very history of Jews marrying other Jews that is seen to be responsible for the increased risk of genetic breast cancer and other diseases. This can lead to a dilemma – marry someone Jewish and risk passing on the disease genes or marry out and risk losing future generations of Jews. The majority of individuals did not suggest marrying non-Jews as a way to reduce the future incidence of disease and appeared to feel a greater sense of responsibility to maintain future generations through both biological (i.e. being 'born Jewish') and social (i.e. upbringing) mechanisms. However, for a small minority of women with strong family histories of genetic disease the solution was for Jews to marry out, or at least to marry a non-Ashkenazi Jew. For these women, genetic responsibility to produce healthy breast-cancer-free children outweighed any potential responsibility for producing future generations of Jews through endogamy.

Rapp (2000: 307) refers to the women she encountered who were making decisions regarding abortion as a result of amniocentesis as 'moral pioneers'. These moral pioneers thought very carefully and underwent substantial emotional, interpersonal and ethical struggles regarding their choices. They enunciated 'a nuanced ethic of reproductive control' (Rapp 2000: 307) as they weighed the burdens of a potentially disabled child against their present demands of motherhood. The women with family histories presented here did feel a responsibility to make reproductive choices that could decrease the risk of breast cancer for their daughters, and for some this responsibility extended in a more subtle and nuanced way to future generations of Jews as a whole. In discussing Dor Yeshorim, Prainsack and Siegal (2006: 17) claim that it creates an atypical concept of genetic responsibility by only revealing 'genetic compatibility' between partners. As a result, a notion of 'genetic couplehood' arises and genetic identity is seen as the joint fate of a couple and bypasses the level of individual awareness of risk. The women described here were expressing individual concern and a sense of genetic responsibility for their own daughters' risk, while also experiencing a responsibility that bypasses the individual or familial and extends more broadly to Jews as a whole. Individual, familial and collective responsibilities are experienced simultaneously.

Importantly, women did not distinguish between the dominant transmission of BRCA mutations and recessive disorders, as evidenced by beliefs about inheriting BRCA mutations from both parents or 'marrying out' as a potential way of decreasing risk. This suggests that an individual's familiarity with Tay-Sachs and screening programmes for recessive diseases has an impact on how genetic breast cancer transmission is understood. Every woman interviewed had heard of Tay-Sachs and was aware that testing was possible, although not all had undergone testing or knew what the disease actually was. While marrying out might help reduce the population risk of BRCA mutations for future generations, it cannot reduce the risk for the individual child (ren) of a mutation carrier. Rather, 'marrying out' appears to be a strategy that simultaneously allocates responsibility for genetic disease onto Ashkenazi Jews as a whole and mitigates women's personal responsibility for passing on mutations to their own children. Women presented themselves as genetically responsible selves but selves that behave responsibly with regard to the future without being held culpable for the past (Hallowell et al. 2006: 983). This suggests that existing knowledge of genetic disease and screening programmes can influence how individuals interpret new genetic knowledge, and there may be potential reproductive consequences and choices may be made on the basis of such (mis)understanding.

Conclusion

When I began this research, I wanted to understand how Ashkenazi women experienced being at increased risk of genetic breast cancer and to know whether this risk made a difference to how they felt about being Jewish, about research related to them, and their disease. My experience working in BRCA clinical research since 2002, especially on Ashkenazi Jewish projects, had shown me that the Ashkenazi Jewish population is utilized frequently, and figures prominently, in this research. Like so many other social scientists, I had the 'reflex suspicion' (Rose 2007: 183) that research specific to a particular racial and ethnic group would be problematic in some way. Surely individuals would be apprehensive about discrimination or stigmatization, or perhaps on a more subtle level feel a sense of unease at being singled out as members of the Ashkenazi Jewish population. I assumed the discrimination that Ashkenazi Jews faced historically would leave a legacy of anxiety about being the subjects of genetic research. In spite of this, and perhaps paradoxically, Ashkenazi Jews have a history of involvement with genetic research and screening programmes and are the most researched population in relation to genetic disease (Birenbaum Carmeli 2004). As a result of this involvement, they are considered to be knowledgeable and keen to take part in research (Kronn et al. 1998, Lehman et al. 2002, Levin 2003, Rapp 2000). How could this be explained? There seemed to be a discrepancy between the potential for discrimination and genetic racism, on the one hand, and Ashkenazi Jews' apparent support for genetic research, on the other. This was the impetus for the questions addressed in this book.

In the introduction I briefly outlined the history of biological theories of racial difference and showed how racial science has been used to justify discrimination, exclusion, social stratification and various other inequalities in the past, with certain racial and ethnic groups being singled out as biologically inferior. This is particularly relevant for the Ashkenazi Jewish population whose long history of discrimination includes being considered a separate biological race that is inferior and more prone to disease (Gilman 1985, 2003). Unsurprisingly, this historical background also informs the majority of the criticisms regarding current genetic research that identifies population differences in disease and illness. Present day research tends to be understood as a contemporary reincarnation of the racial science of the past, leading to concerns that genetic research could have the same potential for negative consequences, including being used to legitimate inequalities (Rose 2007). When the historical context is taken into account, it is easy to understand why much of the debate regarding genetics, population and disease tends to anticipate that the consequences will be damaging and exclusionary.

While it is important not to neglect the past, critics of contemporary genetic research often use these historical negative consequences as warnings of the risks of pursuing such research currently without including the voices of members of high-risk populations (Braun et al. 2007, Caulfield et al. 2009, Gilman 2006, Obasogie 2009). In order to address this gap, this book has explored the views of Ashkenazi Jews at increased risk of genetic breast cancer and the extent to which they were concerned about discrimination, and whether current research was interpreted as potentially harmful in light of past misuses of genetic research. Although when discussing contemporary medical genetic research, the history of Nazi persecution and discrimination inevitably arose, individuals did not see current research as a continuation of, or return to, previous biological discrimination. In fact, interviewees were not particularly concerned about being discriminated against or labelled as ill. Instead, individuals were supportive of genetic medicine and saw genetic testing and screening as valuable mechanisms to help ensure the health of current and future generations of Jews.

The mobilization of Ashkenazi Jews in relation to Tay-Sachs research and screening described in chapter one is undoubtedly an early form of biosociality (Rabinow 1996) that pre-dates current genetic advancements, and the more recent developments in relation to BRCA mutations described in chapter two can be regarded as a continuation of these earlier biosocial activities. High-risk Ashkenazi Jews have raised funds, campaigned, taken part in research and been actively involved in the search for treatments and the development of screening programmes for genetic breast cancer. BRCA advocacy groups, such as JACOB and Sharsheret, which promote genetic testing and population screening studies have the support of local Jewish organizations and community bodies. According to Novas and Rose (2000: 490), persons defined by genetic disease have an investment in scientists fulfilling their promises and discovering the basis of, and the cure or treatment for, genetic diseases, and the genetically at risk individual becomes 'active in the shaping of the enterprise of science'.

There are multiple factors, including Jewish theology, history, political and cultural concerns, which help to explain this supportive attitude towards genetic medicine. Jewish theology, and the way in which health, medicine and abortion are conceptualized, are compatible with genetics and the use of genetic screening. Other culturally specific concerns include Jewish survival, especially following the loss of six million Jews during the Holocaust, and the rising rates of intermarriage. Political concerns over Israel, and the threat to the Israeli state, also make a large and healthy Jewish population important for justifying and ensuring the continued existence of Israel (Prainsack and

Firestine 2006). Many individuals interviewed expressed disquiet about the decreasing population and the implications of this for maintaining adequate numbers both in Israel and the Diaspora. For some such as Emma, who lost most of her paternal family in the Holocaust, the potential of genetic medicine to keep the population healthy and ensure the continued survival of Jewish children was invaluable. Ashkenazi Jews have been actively involved in research and the development of screening programmes because they are mechanisms that address culturally salient issues such as the health of all Jews and the survival of future generations. This supports the arguments of Cowan (2008: 234) that medical genetics is not an extension of historical eugenics, and that genetic testing and screening must not be viewed in the same light as eugenics in the past or present or seen as eugenics of the future. Rather, Cowan (2008) calls into question the frequently made connection between historical eugenics and current medical genetics and claims that the founders of medical genetics viewed their basic project as the relief of human suffering and not the improvement of the human race. Those who use genetic testing and screening are ultimately engaged in a hopeful endeavour aimed at reducing suffering and allowing healthy children to be born. Importantly, research and screening programmes were 'community based' (Cowan 2008: 147) and almost all those involved, from researchers to participants, were Jewish.

At the same time, genetic research and mutations reiterate various aspects of collective Jewish identity and history, such as common founding ancestors, shared lineage, collective suffering and even the endogamous history of Ashkenazi Jews in Eastern Europe, all of which are simultaneously implicated in the causation of genetic disease. For example, the explanations for the increased risk of genetic disease are related to the specific demographic and migratory history of the Jews and their isolation in the ghettos of Eastern Europe. Each of the three BRCA founder mutations has been correlated with a specific event in Jewish history and become a symbol of shared Jewish suffering. The sociopolitical history of Jews is grafted onto the biological explanations of disease in what Montoya calls 'bioethnic conscription' (2007: 95). As a result, genetic disease becomes easily entangled with Jewish identity and issues that are culturally relevant for Jews, such as their shared history and past suffering (Wailoo and Pemberton 2006). In fact, genetic disease and mutations cannot be separated from the social and cultural history of Ashkenazi Jews, what Marks (2008) calls 'biosocial histories' which include life and historical circumstances.

The development of genetic medicine in relation to Ashkenazi Jews, the proliferation of research, and the knowledge that has been generated about disease are as much a result of the social, historical and political context as of their increased risk of disease. This is not to deny that the Ashkenazi Jewish population has a 'palpable and real' (Finkler 2001: 12) risk of genetic disease; however, genetic medicine and Ashkenazi Jews are mutually constitutive and influence each other in a reciprocal relationship. The overall compatibility that we have seen between various aspects of Jewish culture and genetic medicine is integral not only to the ways in which high-risk women interpreted genetic research and disease but also to the development of medicine itself and burgeoning research. The fact that Jewish demographic history fits perfectly with the founder effect and genetic drift, and that Jewish theology is compatible with genetic medicine, and that individuals have specific concerns regarding survival, and even the availability of blood samples, all help to create a climate in which research can flourish.

Jasanoff's (2004) concept of co-production is especially useful in helping to elucidate how scientific and social practices are simultaneously produced. As Jasanoff points out (2004: 2–3), scientific knowledge is not a transcendent mirror of reality; rather, it both embeds and is embedded in social practices, identities, norms, conventions, discourses, instruments and institutions – in short all the building blocks of what we term the *social*. The concept of co-production also avoids the polarization and separation between 'biological' and 'social' categories or distinctions and instead views each as underwriting the other's existence. Important forceful processes flow not only out of science but also into it, and the citadel walls that are frequently assumed to separate science from the rest of history and society are actually rather porous and leaky (Martin 1998), as is evident in the way genetic medicine has developed in relation to Ashkenazi Jews. This serves as a potent reminder of the fluidity and lack of boundaries between the 'biological' and the 'social', which we have seen throughout this book.

The co-production (Jasanoff 2004) of the biological and the social was again evident in the way in which Jewish identity was conceptualized and the impact that genetic disease knowledge had on Jewish self-identity. It has been claimed that research specific to Jews could result in a privileging of biological identity over other social mechanisms that lead to collective identity and create a biologically essentialized view of identity as inborn, natural and unalterable (Azoulay 2003, Brodwin 2002, Kahn 2005). Reardon (2007: 251) cautions that genetic sampling of populations can end up constituting groups defined by race and nation despite its stated intentions to the contrary and as a result 're-biologize identity along racial and national lines'. According to Finkler (2000), genetics is altering traditional notions of kinship and leading to a resurgence of the biological importance of kin and family in relation to genetic disease. I anticipated that being at increased risk of genetic disease would cause individuals to question their own identity, or perhaps reject the idea that they were members of a biological group. For most individuals I met, genetics did not lead to a transformation in identity or to biologically essentialized thinking about being Jewish. Again, interviewees mentioned the past, especially Nazi persecution, to point out the dangers of being referred to in biological terms but when they talked about their own Jewish identity, biology was an important defining feature, whether in terms of the requirement to be born Jewish, have a Jewish mother or their descent from common ancestors. At the same time, being Jewish was thought of as a cultural identity born out of shared upbringing, religious observance, rituals and social and political concerns. These were not mutually exclusive and this research highlights the complex and multiple ways in which identity can be conceived of by Ashkenazi Jews. In fact, the very meaning of 'social' and 'biological' are called into question, as individuals often did not express a biogenetic understanding of what was biological. For example, while Jewish mothers lead to Jewish children, Jewish fathers do not. But in this understanding, what happens to the biological and genetic material the father has contributed? While some individuals rejected using the word biological to refer to Ashkenazi Jews, they concurrently referred to 'Jewish blood' and birth. Jewish identity is already a combination of the biological and social, yet none of these conceptions of being Jewish map neatly onto categories of 'biological', 'genetic', 'social' or 'cultural'. As Kahn (2000) accurately notes, separating the biological and social is impossible when thinking about Jewish kinship. Concerns that new genetic knowledge will lead to a privileging of biological over cultural identity fail to recognize that identity can very often comprise both, and that biology (however it is defined or experienced) can be a vital way in which people feel linked and connected to one another.

Genetics has the potential to reaffirm the pre-existing ways in which collective identity is conceptualized for Ashkenazi Jews and does not necessarily have a detrimental or problematic effect. According to Novas and Rose (2000: 495), when an individual goes for a genetic consultation, this involves a 'genetic re-mapping where the individual reconfigures their identity in terms of a genetic past, a genetic present and a genetic future'. Reardon (2005: 253) directs our attention to the 'affective ties people form to their new technoscientific identities'. For Ashkenazi Jews, being at increased risk of genetic disease does not necessarily involve a re-mapping, new affective ties or a destabilization of identity; rather, it is fairly consistent with the conception of Jewish belonging that includes a genetic past with descent from common ancestors, a genetic present that sees Jews as interrelated and a genetic future in which the survival of subsequent generations of Jews is critical. Having a shared risk of genetic disease is not a radical break with how most interviewees already conceived of themselves, which confirms Prainsack's (2007) argument that the findings of genetics and biology are consistent with pre-existing ways of thinking about Jewish identity and can help create boundaries that reinforce group belonging. This sense of being part of one large extended 'family' is another factor that creates support for genetic screening programmes and testing because they offer the possibility of altering the health of the entire 'family' of Ashkenazi Jews; individuals sometimes even made references to Jews as a family.

However, Rachel's story described in chapter four did indicate that genetic knowledge has the potential to transform concepts of identity in complicated ways. For Rachel, her increased risk of genetic breast cancer led to uncomfortable questions about the nature of Judaism and whether Jews were a race, which was especially difficult because she did not think of her Jewish identity in a biological way. Although Rachel was the only woman I met who felt this way, her experience suggests that for some people genetics can conflict with, rather than confirm, how they perceive of their belonging, and this is an area that would be worthy of exploration in future research. Importantly, Rachel associated being Jewish with being different and singled out, and not something she especially liked to identify with. Her experience of Judaism was a more stigmatizing one, which contributed to the reason she found it challenging to think of her Jewishness in a biological way because this implied it was unchangeable. Rachel did not derive a lot of personal fulfilment from being Jewish and preferred being able to distance herself from this aspect of her identity. In contrast, the other individuals interviewed did not describe their Jewish identities in this way, even though some had faced anti-Semitism or felt set apart because of their Jewishness. For most, being Jewish created a sense of connection and comfort from which they obtained various personal benefits and as a result it was less problematic to consider themselves as members of a biological group, and easier to accept genetic disease as one unfortunate aspect of their belonging. This illustrates how individual experiences of ethnicity and collective belonging, especially in terms of stigmatization or exclusion, can be important contributing factors to how genetic knowledge is interpreted. The impact of new genetic knowledge on identity can be contingent upon the positive or negative associations individuals have with their own ethnicity. Examining many perspectives is important for understanding race and ethnicity in the genomics era (Nelson 2008) and any claims must take into account the complex and varied ways in which specific populations and individuals conceptualize their identity.

It is important to note that this research provides information about the concerns, or lack thereof, that a sample of well-educated Ashkenazi Jewish individuals living in London had about genetic research and disease, and the implications of genetic disease knowledge on Jewish self-identity, but it does not provide information regarding how non-Jews and other Jews in different contexts may interpret the same knowledge. However, the aim of this research was to give life to the voices of members of high-risk populations, which are often not included in research, while recognizing this is only one piece of the larger picture. In addition, the majority of the women interviewed were secular and not religiously observant and no ultra-Orthodox Jews were interviewed. These women are not representative of 'Ashkenazi Jews' or Jewish views, and the ways in which more religious or ultra-Orthodox women might have experienced their increased risk of genetic breast cancer, or being the subjects of genetic research, remain unknown. It is also possible that there are Ashkenazi individuals who refuse genetic services or testing because they are uncomfortable with them, and one area of future research would be to investigate the reasons for such refusal. Kahn (2005) suggests that biological reasoning about Jewish belonging may be particularly appealing for those whose sense of Jewishness is not a result of commitment to the ritual laws and customs of Judaism, and interviewees repeatedly described their Jewishness as not being the product of ritual observance. Importantly, this lack of ritual observance did not affect individuals' sense of still 'feeling very Jewish' or prevent them from identifying themselves as Jews, which confirms that commitment to religious practice is not the primary factor upon which secular Jews base their identity. More observant or ultra-Orthodox Jews might feel very differently about both what defines their belonging and the implications of having genetic disease as a result, and this is another potential area for future research.

Does this mean that many of the concerns raised about genetic research, in particular that Jews will be labelled as ill or that it will result in an increase in discrimination, are unfounded? There is not a straightforward answer to this question, and there was evidence that doctors, clinical encounters, family history questionnaires and population screening projects at times left women with an exaggerated belief that all Ashkenazi women are at increased risk of genetic breast cancer. This demonstrates how the increased risk for a group can easily become confused with an increased risk for all individuals within that group, and even doctors sometimes inaccurately had this impression, which they relayed to their patients. While this misconception was not problematic for the women I interviewed, who were more concerned with raising awareness, it could potentially lead to an increase in stigmatization or discrimination by others. This research explored the perspective of Jewish women on this topic, but an important area for future research would be to examine how non-Jews interpret Jews' higher risk and whether they think of Jews as being more prone to genetic disease and other illnesses.

The knowledge of being at increased genetic risk of breast cancer was not without consequences and led to considerable anxiety for women, as described especially in chapters five and six. During interviews and clinical appointments, women expressed significant worries about the possibility of developing breast cancer or a recurrence in future, making decisions about screening and prophylactic surgery, and the uncertainty of negative test results despite having strong family histories. There were stories of silence, secrecy and denial in respect of family histories of breast cancer, and indications of possible guilt about being a carrier and passing genetic mutations to children. This is a stark reminder of the consequences of genetic knowledge about breast cancer risk and testing more broadly. There was also evidence of women undergoing genetic testing for the sake of their daughters, even when they were unsure if they wanted the information themselves. The 'right not to know' may not be realizable for women who feel an obligation to get genetic testing for the sake of others, and in particular their daughters or mothers (Hallowell 1999). Kenen (1996) refers to the assumption that knowledge is intrinsically good and enables informed decision making as the 'gift of knowing'. However, knowledge is not always a gift and women expressed ambivalence about the value of BRCA mutation testing and the information that would arise from it.

Chapter six demonstrated that genetics is a powerful tool that can lead to a sense of genetic responsibility (Hallowell 1999, Novas and Rose 2000) to take certain actions in relation to ourselves, our family, our children and, importantly for Ashkenazi Jews, to the entire broader 'community'. Women located responsibility for genetic disease in the collective endogamous history of Ashkenazi Jews. Again, collective history (in terms of endogamy) is implicated in the causation of disease, while at the same time disease reiterates collective history (in terms of endogamy). In the present, women allocated blame and responsibility to the ultra-Orthodox, who were seen as possibly perpetuating genetic disease due to their high birth rate, and the possibility of consanguineous marriages. At the same time, endogamy remains important to many Ashkenazi Jews, who feel a responsibility to marry other Jews in order to ensure the survival of future generations. However, the knowledge that genetic disease is a result of endogamous marriage may come into conflict with this imperative. The majority of individuals did not suggest marrying non-Jews as a way to reduce the future incidence of disease and appeared to feel a greater sense of responsibility to maintain future generations through both biological (i.e. being 'born Jewish') and social (i.e. upbringing) mechanisms. However, for some women with strong family histories of genetic disease 'marrying out' was a strategy that they proposed to reduce the risk of genetic breast cancer in future generations. The suggestion to marry out was a reflection of women's concerns for their own daughters' risk, while it also displaced responsibility for genetic disease onto Jews as a whole, which may have helped to minimize individual responsibility for passing on mutations. Importantly, women did not distinguish between dominant and recessive transmission patterns. Familiarity with Tay-Sachs screening, and its recessive transmission, led some women to assume that marrying out would reduce the risk of their daughters developing BRCA genetic breast cancer. Unfortunately for women who are mutation carriers, their own daughters' risk remains the same regardless of their choice of marriage partner. Previous knowledge of genetic disease and screening programmes, such as those for Tay-Sachs, can influence how individuals interpret new genetic knowledge, and there may be potential reproductive consequences and choices based on such (mis)understanding. This is another indication of the strong sense of genetic responsibility that can result from having a family history of breast cancer, with individual, familial and collective responsibilities being experienced simultaneously.

BRCA mutation testing is a routinized clinical procedure and Ashkenazi women are frequently referred to clinics and advised to undergo testing, which is consistent with the UK national clinical guidelines (National Institute of Clinical Excellence 2005). Genetic counsellors reported offering testing more often to Ashkenazi patients even when there was not a particularly strong family history; thus Ashkenazi Jewish patients may face a lower threshold for being offered testing when compared to other individuals. Although clinicians and nurses warned women about the drawbacks of testing, this did not eliminate many of the difficult issues they faced. While expressing a generally supportive and positive attitude towards genetic knowledge, it is essential not to ignore the significant emotional and psychological consequences such knowledge of risk can have for individual women and their families. The fact that some clinicians believed Ashkenazi Jews were more prone to disease could lead to unnecessary genetics referrals and possibly genetic tests, and it is important to think about the impact this may have on women. For example, Susan was offered, and underwent, genetic testing after her first clinical appointment, but when we met she had changed her mind about wanting the results. Susan's genetic counsellor was unaware of this and explained to me that Ashkenazi patients had a tendency to demand the test without wanting a great deal of discussion. There is a danger that Ashkenazi women may be offered testing too easily and without being given adequate time to consider the long-term implications, and this research highlights the potential consequences of making generalizations or assumptions about specific populations. While the experiences of the women presented here may not be unique to Ashkenazi Jews, it is important to bear in mind that if Ashkenazi women are identified in clinical encounters and referred to genetic counselling more frequently, then they may face these emotional and psychological consequences more often.

Ashkenazi Jews are an iconic example of a population that has become over-represented in medical genetics, something which has had both benefits and drawbacks. They have benefited in terms of screening programmes and a reduction in the frequency of disease (mostly recessive diseases), while there have been drawbacks such as ever increasing knowledge about 'Jewish diseases' despite the fact that little is known about disease incidence in other populations. The scientific knowledge about the increased risk of genetic breast cancer was derived from samples that were donated by those taking part in Tay-Sachs research and screening in the early 1970s, and research has continued to build on this pre-existing body of literature and samples (Wailoo and Pemberton 2006). Although Ashkenazi Jews have willingly continued to donate further samples for research, participating in genetic research studies can result in ever increasing and self-perpetuating knowledge about certain populations, while other groups may remain under-represented.

This also raises questions about representation in genetic research and medicine more broadly. In particular, those who are under-represented may not derive the potential benefits of genetic medicine, especially as there are increasing efforts to develop personalized medicine, that is, medicine based on individual or population genetic profiling. For example, in the United States, African Americans and Hispanics are insufficiently represented in BRCA clinical services and testing (as well as many other health care arenas). This under-representation has worsened health disparities, and researchers are concerned that the lack of data on particular populations may make the available data less relevant. This has led to programmes specifically aimed at increasing referrals and recruitment of members of these populations to clinical and research services (Mozersky and Joseph 2010). Research is under way to determine BRCA mutation frequencies in African Americans and Hispanic/Latino Americans (Olopade 2004, Olopade et al. 2005, Weitzel et al. 2005, 2007). In Brazil, a high incidence of 'Ashkenazi founder mutations' has also been discovered in families with a history of breast cancer (da Costa et al. 2008), raising questions about whether these mutations should be designated 'Ashkenazi Jewish' at all.

The findings of this research are therefore important not only for the population of Ashkenazi Jews which is its subject but also for the broader debate about genetic research on populations. For the Ashkenazi Jews in this study, knowing the genetic basis of disease is a way to increase the possibility of effective intervention, improve the health of the population, and ensure the survival of future generations. Genetic medicine is therefore allying itself with the demands and concerns of this biosocial community and addressing culturally specific needs (Rose 2007: 183). This may be more important than concerns about discrimination or being singled out and labelled as ill, but whether this would be true of populations with a different historical or social context remains an unanswered question. It cannot be assumed that the supportive attitude expressed by individuals in this study will be reflected by other Ashkenazi Jews or in other populations, and it is essential to investigate the specific sociocultural and national contexts of different ethnoracial groups before drawing any conclusions about how genetic research will be received and interpreted. For example, in France the universalist conception of citizenship does not favour focusing on ethnic issues in general or in relation to breast cancer, and ethnicity and Ashkenazi Jewish origin are not significantly associated with breast cancer (Lowy and Gaudilliere 2008). Similarly, women in the UK can access genetic testing for BRCA mutations free of charge through the National Health Service, whereas the commercial monopoly on BRCA testing held by Myriad in the United States has resulted in an entirely different 'architecture' of genetic testing with unequal access and a high cost of testing (Parthasarathy 2007).

According to Nelson (2008), the longings of members of racial or ethnic groups undergoing genetic testing, whether in relation to disease or to uncover genealogical roots, are often shaped by histories of oppression. The sense of empowerment and autonomy gained from genetic knowledge may come at the cost of acquiescing to a classificatory logic of human racial and ethnic differences that compounds, rather than challenges, social inequality (Nelson 2008: 776). Ashkenazi Jews are shaped by a history of oppression and participate in genetic research because it empowers them to take control of their health and that of the entire population, but this may simultaneously magnify concepts of Jewish difference and ill health. The results of this research indicate that it is not necessary to begin from a highly critical or suspicious stance regarding population, race/ethnicity, genetics and disease, and there are clearly potential benefits to be gained for those populations who acquire knowledge about diseases as a result of current research. However, genetic research may lead to renewed associations with disease, generalizations about all Ashkenazi Jews, increased clinical referrals and even possible discrimination, and it is essential that we continue to monitor and contextualize these developments as they pertain to specific populations.

Notes

Introduction

1 Although Birenbaum Carmeli's (2004) method of calculating citations in the literature has some limitations, Ashkenazi Jews are more represented than any other population group in scientific genetic disease literature.
2 Marks (2002) has questioned the significance of such figures given that humans and chimps are 98 per cent similar genetically, and the functional significance of the majority of the human genome is estimated to be only 1–2 per cent.
3 Some examples include the NIH Pharmacogenetics Research Network, the NIH Centre on Genomics and Health Disparities, the failed Human Genome Diversity Project and the Genographic project.
4 http://www.1000genomes.org/about (online, accessed 12 December 2011).
5 There are qualitative studies that examine how scientists and researchers use race and ethnicity in their research (see Montoya 2007 and Fullwiley 2007 for examples), but these studies tend not to include the voices or views of the populations being researched. Prainsack (2007) and Kahn (2000) interviewed Jewish women and men in Israel about their views of reproductive technologies but did not specifically address concerns regarding discrimination in relation to genetic disease, or the impact on identity. Nelson (2008) explored the implications of genetic genealogy knowledge, rather than genetic disease, on concepts of racial identity for African Americans and Black British consumers of genealogy tests.
6 For aesthetic reasons I have not put social and biological in quotation marks throughout the text, although I recognize the ambiguity and lack of boundaries when using these terms. I occasionally put them in quotes when I am particularly trying to draw attention to this ambiguity.

1 Setting the scene: Ashkenazi Jews and genetic disease

1 Genes occur in pairs, with one copy coming from the mother and the other from the father. A single member of the pair is an allele.
2 In contrast to Ashkenazi Jews, Sephardi Jews are those who left the Middle East and settled primarily in Spain. The term Sephardi also includes their descendants wherever they resided, as the Jews of Spain were expelled in 1492 and many settled along the North African coast and in Italy, Egypt, Palestine and Syria (Goodman 1979). Mizrahi (or Oriental) Jews are those who remained in the Middle East, including Israel, Iraq, Iran and other surrounding regions. Mizrahi Jews represent the 'original gene pool' of all Jews, while Sephardi and Ashkenazi Jews are those who left this region and became various Diasporas (Goldstein 2008). The migrational and geographic separation of Ashkenazi, Sephardic and Mizrahi Jews resulted in genetic differentiation and illustrates the way in which genetic variation is a reflection of the geographical, migration and reproductive histories of particular groups.

3 http://www.jewishgeneticdiseases.org/ (online, accessed 12 January 2012).
4 Having a bar or bat (for girls) mitzvah was an important way in which people I interviewed identified themselves as Jews. I always asked individuals to tell me about their personal Jewish upbringing and they most often used whether or not they had a bar or bat mitzvah as an indicator of whether their upbringing was 'Jewish' or not. Even people who did not describe themselves as having a particularly Jewish upbringing very often had had bar or bat mitzvahs. One woman who had not had a bat mitzvah was considering taking Hebrew lessons and having a bat mitzvah as an adult to make up for the sense of loss she felt at not having had one as an adolescent.
5 See Gessen (2008) and Raz (2010) for detailed and fascinating examinations of how Dor Yeshorim actually operates among individual ultra-Orthodox Jewish families
6 In the controversial Tuskegee experiments, African American men with syphilis were studied to determine the effects of syphilis in the absence of any treatment. They were given a fake ointment so that they believed they were receiving treatment and many of the volunteers died of syphilis (Duster 1990).
7 Embryos that are outside the uterus, for example as a result of in vitro fertilization (IVF), are not even regarded as comparable in any way to an implanted embryo, which also contributes to the high acceptance and use of reproductive technologies in Israel (Prainsack and Firestine 2006, Rosner 2001).

2 The 'Ashkenazi BRCA mutations'

1 Israeli collaborators did not actually anticipate putting in any more patients than clinicians in other countries.
2 A polymorphism is a particular sequence of DNA that is passed from generation to generation and does not necessarily cause disease or have any disadvantage.
3 http://www.geneticalliance.org/about (online, accessed 12 January 2012).
4 Until October 2009, the UK Human Fertilisation and Embryology Authority (HFEA) decided on the permissibility of PGD for BRCA mutations on a case by case basis. Prior to October 2009, there were fewer than 10 applications made by centres to carry out PGD for BRCA. Since October 2009, the majority of conditions, including BRCA testing, are licensed on an 'in principle' basis, which means that if the licensing committee approves the use of PGD for a particular condition by a specific laboratory, then this laboratory can carry out PGD for that condition without applying for each use on a case by case basis. http://www.hfea.gov.uk/6035.html (online, accessed 20 January 2012).
5 http://www.instituteforwomenshealth.ucl.ac.uk/academic_research/gynaecologicalcancer/gcrc/gcapps (online, accessed 20 January 2012).

4 On being Jewish

1 Thank you to Barbara Prainsack for pointing this out and helping me to elucidate this point.
2 http://www.jewishvirtuallibrary.org/jsource/US-Israel/usjewpop.html (online, accessed 20 January 2012).
3 http://video.nytimes.com/video/2007/08/31/health/1194817106561/the-story-of-a-previvor.html (online, accessed 6 January 2012).
4 I sometimes felt that the genetic counsellors made more of an effort to explain and discuss the Ashkenazi mutations when I was sitting in on the clinic appointments.

5 History, memory and the BRCA genes

1 © 2001 by the Wenner-Gren Foundation for Anthropological Research. All rights reserved.

2 I asked Nancy directly if this had made her more worried and she told me that it had made her a 'little bit' more worried when she was reminded of this risk. This made me concerned that my own research was creating anxiety among Ashkenazi Jewish women, which was something I had been eager to avoid before the research began. However, these were the only two occasions where I encountered women who were made aware or reminded of the increased risk because of my study.

3 Proctor (1999) discusses the ways in which Nazi science stimulated a great deal of research into the causes of cancer that is often not publicized. Beyond heritability, there was research into the environmental causes of cancer during this period. Proctor suggests that while we may be reluctant to acknowledge it, many public health policies implemented by the Nazis would be considered socially responsible today. This included policies to promote the importance of a diet free from petrochemical dyes and preservatives, the consumption of whole grain foods, vegetarianism and a concern with animal welfare as well as anti-smoking campaigns. According to Proctor, Nazism was popular not just because of anti-Semitism but also because it offered people many public health promises.

6 Future generations

1 There are support groups specifically for ultra-Orthodox mothers of disabled children. In London there is a group called 'In Touch'.

2 This experience was something I was personally familiar with, as I had grown up with many Jewish friends whose parents had strictly forbidden their children from dating non-Jews.

References

Abbott, A. (2005) 'Genetic patent singles out Jewish women', *Nature*, 436 (7047): 12.

Agar, N. (2004) *Liberal Eugenics in Defence of Human Enhancement*, Oxford: Wiley-Blackwell Publishing.

Angier, N. (1994) 'Vexing pursuit of breast cancer gene', *New York Times*, Science section, 12 July 1994.

Antoniou, A.C., Gayther, S.A., Stratton, J.F., Ponder, B.A. and Easton, D.F. (2000) 'Risk models for familial ovarian and breast cancer', *Genetic Epidemiology,* 18 (2): 173 90.

Antoniou, A.C., Pharoah, P.D.P., Narod, S., Risch, H.A., Eyfjord, J.E., Hopper, J.L., Loman, N., Olsson, H., Johannsson, O., Borg, A., Pasini, B., Radice, P., Manoukian, S., Eccles, D.M., Tang, N., Olah, E., Anton-Culver, H., Warner, E., Lubinski, J., Gronwald, J., Gorski, B., Tulinius, H., Thorlacius, S., Eerola, H., Nevanlinna, H., Syrjkoski, K., Kallioniemi, O.P., Thompson, D., Evans, C., Peto, J., Lalloo, F., Evans, D.G. and Easton, D.F. (2003) 'Average risks of breast and ovarian cancer associated with BRCA1 or BRCA2 mutations detected in case series unselected for family history: a combined analysis of 22 studies', *American Journal of Human Genetics*, 72 (5): 1117–30.

Arcos, B. (2002) 'Genetics of population isolates', *Clinical Genetics*, (61) 4: 233–47.

Arribas-Ayllon, M., Sarangi, S. and Clarke, A. (2008a) 'Managing self-responsibility through other-oriented blame: family accounts of genetic testing', *Social Science & Medicine*, 66 (7): 1521–32.

Arribas-Ayllon, M., Sarangi, S. and Clarke, A. (2008b) 'The micropolitics of responsibility vis-à-vis autonomy: parental accounts of childhood genetic testing and (non)disclosure', *Sociology of Health & Illness*, 30 (2): 255–71.

Azoulay, K.G. (2003) 'Not an innocent pursuit: the politics of a "jewish" genetic signature', *Developing World Bioethics* (3) 2: 119–26.

Azoulay, K.G. (2006) 'Reflections on "race" and the biologization of difference', *Patterns of Prejudice*, 40 (4–5): 353–79.

Balmaña, J., Domchek, S.M., Tutt, A. and Garber, J.E. (2011) 'Stumbling blocks on the path to personalized medicine in breast cancer: the case of PARP inhibitors for BRCA1/2-associated cancers', *Cancer Discovery*, 1(1): 29.

Bamshad, M., Wooding, S., Salisbury, B.A. and Stephens, J.C. (2004) 'Deconstructing the relationship between genetics and race', *Nature Review Genetics*, 5 (8): 598–609.

Bankhead, C., Richards, S.H., Peters, T.J., Sharp, D.J., Hobbs, F.D.R., Brown, J., Roberts, L., Tydeman, C., Redman, V., Formby, J., Wilson, S. and Austoker, J. (2001) 'Improving attendance for breast screening among recent non-attenders: a randomised controlled trial of two interventions in primary care', *Journal of Medical Screening*, 8: 99–105.

Bar-Sade, R.B., Kruglikova, A., Modan, B., Gak, E., Hirsh-Yechezkel, G., Theodor, L., Novikov, I., Gershoni-Baruch, R., Risel, S., Papa, M.Z., Ben-Baruch, G. and Friedman, E. (1998) 'The 185delAG BRCA1 mutation originated before the dispersion of Jews in the Diaspora and is not limited to Ashkenazim', *Human Molecular Genetics*, 7 (5): 801–5.

Behar, D.M., Metspalu, E., Kivisild, T., Achilli, A., Hadid, Y., Tzur, S., Pereira, L., Amorim, A., Quintana-Murci, L., Majamaa, K., Herrnstadt, C., Howell, N., Balanovsky, O., Kutuev, I., Pshenichnov, A., Gurwitz, D., Bonne-Tamir, B., Torroni, A., Villems, R. and Skorecki, K. (2006) 'The matrilineal ancestry of Ashkenazi Jewry: portrait of a recent founder event', *American Journal of Human Genetics*, 78 (3): 487–97.

Berman, L.C. (2010) 'Blame, boundaries and birthrights', pp. 91–110 in S.A. Glenn and N.B. Sokoloff (eds) *Boundaries of Jewish Identity*, Seattle, WA: University of Washington Press.

Birenbaum Carmeli, D. (2004) 'Prevalence of Jews as subjects in genetic research: figures, explanation, and potential implications', *American Journal of Medical Genetics*, 130A: 76–83.

Bittles, A.H. (2005) 'Endogamy, consanguinity and community disease profiles', *Public Health Genomics*, 8 (1): 17–20.

Bradby, H. (1996) 'Genetics and racism', pp. 295–316 in T. Marteau and M. Richards (eds) *The Troubled Helix: Social and Psychological Implications of the New Human Genetics*, Cambridge: Cambridge University Press.

Braun, L., Fausto-Sterling, A., Fullwiley, D., Hammonds, E.M., Nelson, A., Quivers, W., Reverby, S.M. and Shields, A.E. (2007) 'Racial categories in medical practice: how useful are they?', *PLoS Medicine*, 4 (9): e271.

Breast Cancer Action (2011) Online, http://thinkbeforeyoupink.org/ (accessed 5 January 2012).

Broadstock, M., Michie, S. and Marteau, T. (2000) 'Psychological consequences of predictive genetic testing: a systematic review', *European Journal of Human Genetics*, 8 (10): 731–8.

Brodwin, P. (2002) 'Genetics, identity, and the anthropology of essentialism', *Anthropological Quarterly*, 75 (2): 323–30.

Burchard, E.G., Ziv, E., Coyle, N., Lin-Gomez, S., Tang, H., Karter, A.J., Mountain, J., Perez-Stable, E.J., Sheppard, D. and Risch, N. (2003) 'The importance of race and ethnic background in biomedical research and clinical practice', *New England Journal of Medicine*, 348 (12): 1077–92.

Byrne, B. (2004) 'Qualitative interviewing', pp. 179–92 in C. Seale (ed.) *Researching Society and Culture*, London: Sage.

Cancer Research UK (2008) 'Cancer stats incidence'. Online, http://info.cancerresearchuk.org/cancerstats/types/ovary/ (accessed 22 December 2011).

Casper, M. and Koenig, B. (1996) 'Reconfiguring nature and culture: intersections of medical anthropology and technoscience studies', *Medical Anthropology Quarterly*, 10 (4): 523–36.

Caulfield, T., Fullerton, S.M., Ali-Khan, S.E., Arbour, L., Burchard, E.G., Cooper, R. S., Hardy, B.J., Harry, S., Hyde-Lay, R., Kahn, J., Kittles, R., Koenig, B.A., Lee, S. J., Malinowski, M., Ravitsky, V., Sankar, P., Scherer, S.W., Séguin, B., Shickle, D., Suarez-Kurtz, G. and Daar Abdallah, S. (2009) 'Race and ancestry in biomedical research: exploring the challenges', *Genome Medicine*, 1 (1): article 8.

Clow, B. (2001) 'Who's afraid of Susan Sontag? Or the myths and metaphors of cancer reconsidered', *Social History of Medicine*, 14 (2): 293–312.

Cochran, G., Hardy, J. and Harpending, H. (2005) 'Natural history of Ashkenazi intelligence', *Journal of Biosocial Science*, 38 (5): 659–93.

Collins, F. (2004) 'What we do and don't know about "race", "ethnicity", genetics and health at the dawn of the genome area', *Nature Genetics*, 36 (11): S13–15, November supplement.

Connerton, P. (1989) *How Societies Remember*, Cambridge: Cambridge University Press.

Cowan, R.S. (2008) *Heredity and Hope: The Case for Genetic Screening*, Cambridge, MA: Harvard University Press.

Cox, S. and McKellin, W. (1999) 'There's this thing in our family: predictive testing and the construction of risk for Huntington's disease', pp. 121–48 in P. Conrad and J. Gabe (eds) *Sociological Perspectives on the New Genetics*, Oxford: Blackwell Publishing.

Croyle, R.T., Smith, K.R., Botkin, J.R., Baty, B. and Nash, J. (1997) 'Psychological responses to BRCA1 mutation testing: preliminary findings', *Health Psychology*, 16 (1): 63–72.

da Costa, E.C.B., Vargas, F.R., Moreira, A.S., Lourenço, J.J., Caletti, M., Ashton-Prolla, P. and Martins Moreira, M.A. (2008) 'Founder effect of the BRCA1 5382insC mutation in Brazilian patients with hereditary breast ovary cancer syndrome', *Cancer Genetics and Cytogenetics*, 184 (1): 62–6.

Dein, S. (2002) 'Mosiach is here now: just open your eyes and you can see him', *Anthropology & Medicine*, 9 (1): 25–36.

Donelle, L., Hoffman-Goetz, L. and Clarke, J.N. (2005) 'Ethnicity, genetics, and breast cancer: media portrayal of disease identities', *Ethnicity & Health*, 10 (3): 185–97.

Dorff, R.E.N. (1997) 'Jewish theological and moral reflections on genetic screening: the case of BRCA1', *Health Matrix: Journal of Law-Medicine*, 7: 65–96.

Durfy, S.J., Bowen, D.J., McTiernan, A., Sporleder, J. and Burke, W. (1999) 'Attitudes and interest in genetic testing for breast and ovarian cancer susceptibility in diverse groups of women in western Washington', *Cancer Epidemiology, Biomarkers & Prevention*, 8 (4): 369–75.

Duster, T. (1990) *Backdoor to Eugenics*, New York: Routledge.

Duster, T. (2005) 'Medicine enhanced: race and reification in science', *Science*, 307 (5712): 1050–1.

Duster, T. (2006) 'The molecular reinscription of race: unanticipated issues in biotechnology and forensic science', *Patterns of Prejudice*, 40 (4–5): 427–41.

Edelson, P.J. (1997) 'The Tay Sachs disease screening program in the US as a model for the control of genetic disease: an historical overview', *Health Matrix: Journal of Law-Medicine*, 7: 125–33.

Edwards, J. and Strathern, M. (2000) 'Including our own', pp. 149–66 in J. Carsten (ed.) *Cultures of Relatedness: New Approaches to the Study of Kinship*, Cambridge: Cambridge University Press.

Ekstein, J. and Katzenstein, H. (2001) 'The Dor Yeshorim story: community-based carrier screening for Tay-Sachs disease', *Advances in Genetics*, 44: 297–310.

Ellison, G.T.H., Smart, A., Tutton, R., Outram, S.M., Ashcroft, R. and Martin, P. (2007) 'Racial categories in medicine: a failure of evidence-based practice?', *PLoS Medicine*, 4 (9): e287.

Endelman, T.M. (2004) 'Anglo-Jewish scientists and the science of race', *Jewish Social Studies*, 11 (1): 52–92.

Epstein, S. (2007) *Inclusion: The Politics of Difference in Medical Research*, Chicago, IL: University of Chicago Press.

Finkler, K. (2000) *Experiencing the New Genetics: Family and Kinship on the Medical Frontier*, Philadelphia: University of Pennsylvania Press.

Finkler, K. (2001) 'The kin in the gene – the medicalization of family and kinship in American society', *Current Anthropology*, 42 (2): 235–63.

Fletcher, R. (2007) 'Funding boost for cancer gene expert', *Jewish Chronicle*, 23 March 2007: 14.

Foster, M.W. and Sharp, R.R. (2002) 'Race, ethnicity, and genomics: social classifications as proxies of biological heterogeneity', *Genome Research*, 12 (6): 844–50.

Foucault, M. (1988) 'The ethic of care for the self as a practice of freedom, an interview with Michel Foucault on January 20, 1984', pp. 1–20 in J. Bernauer and D. Rasmussen (eds) *The Final Foucault*, Cambridge, MA: MIT Press.

Franklin, S. (1995) 'Science as culture, cultures of science', *Annual Review of Anthropology*, 24: 163–84.

Franklin, S. (2003) 'Re-thinking nature–culture', *Anthropological Theory*, 3 (1): 65–85.

Friedman, L. (2010) 'Intermarriage spurs Tay-Sachs advisory', *Jewish Daily Forward*. Online, http://www.forward.com/articles/129987/ (accessed 22 December 2011).

Fujimura, J.H. (1996) *Crafting Science: A Sociohistory of the Quest for the Genetics of Cancer*, Cambridge, MA: Harvard University Press.

Fujimura, J.H., Duster, T. and Rajagopalan, R. (2008) 'Introduction: race, genetics, and disease: questions of evidence, matters of consequence', *Social Studies of Science*, 38 (5): 643–56.

Fullwiley, D. (2007) 'Race and genetics: attempts to define the relationship', *BioSocieties*, 2 (2): 221–37.

Fullwiley, D. (2008) 'The biologistical construction of race: "admixture" technology and the new genetic medicine', *Social Studies of Science*, 38 (5): 695–735.

Galton, F. (1883) *Inquiries into Human Faculty and Its Development*, London: Dent & Co. Online, http://galton.org/ (accessed 9 January 2012).

Gessen, M. (2008) *Blood Matters: A Journey along the Genetic Frontier*, London: Granta Books.

Gibbon, S. and Novas, C. (eds) (2007) *Biosocialities, Identity and the Social Sciences*, London: Routledge.

Gilman, S.L. (1985) *Difference and Pathology: Stereotypes of Sexuality, Race and Madness*, Ithaca, NY: Cornell University Press.

Gilman, S.L. (2003) *Jewish Frontiers: Essays on Bodies, Histories and Identities*, New York: Palgrave Macmillan.

Gilman, S.L. (2006) 'Genetic diseases? Yes. But must we call them Jewish?', *Jewish Daily Forward*. Online, http://www.forward.com/articles/1471/ (accessed 13 January 2012).

Glenn, S.A. (2010) 'Funny, you don't look Jewish', pp. 64–91 in S.A. Glenn and N.B. Sokoloff (eds) *Boundaries of Jewish Identity*, Seattle, WA: University of Washington Press.

Glenn, S.A. and Sokoloff, N.B. (eds) (2010) *Boundaries of Jewish Identity*, Seattle, WA: University of Washington Press.

Goldstein, D.B. (2008) *Jacob's Legacy: A Genetic View of Jewish History*, New Haven, CT: Yale University Press.

Goodman, A.H., Heath, D. and Lindee, M.S. (eds) (2003) *Genetic Nature/Culture: Anthropology and Science beyond the Two-Culture Divide*, Berkeley, CA: University of California Press.

Goodman, M.J. and Goodman, L.E. (1982) 'The overselling of genetic anxiety', *Hastings Center Report*, 12 (5): 20–7.

Goodman, R.M. (1979) *Genetic Disorders among the Jewish People*, Baltimore, MD: Johns Hopkins University Press.

Gould, S.J. (1981) *The Mismeasure of Man*, New York: W.W. Norton & Company.

Graham, D. (2004) 'European Jewish identity at the dawn of the 21st century: a working paper. A report prepared for the American Jewish Joint Distribution Committee and Hanadiv Charitable Foundation'. Presented to the European General Assembly of the European Council of Jewish Communities, Budapest, 20–23 May 2004. Online, http://www.jpr.org.uk/sitemap.php (accessed 30 October 2011).

Grann, V.R., Whang, W., Jacobson, J.S., Heitjan, D.F., Antman, K.H. and Neugut, A.I. (1999) 'Benefits and costs of screening Ashkenazi Jewish women for BRCA1 and BRCA2', *Journal of Clinical Oncology*, 17 (2): 494.

Haber, D. (2002) 'Prophylactic oophorectomy to reduce the risk of ovarian and breast cancer in carriers of BRCA mutations', *New England Journal of Medicine*, 346 (21): 1660–62.

Hallowell, N. (1999) 'Doing the right thing: genetic risk and responsibility', pp. 97–119 in P. Conrad and J. Gabe (eds) *Sociological Perspectives on the New Genetics*, Oxford: Blackwell Publishing.

Hallowell, N., Murton, F., Statham, H., Green, J.M. and Richards, M.P.M. (1997) 'Women's need for information before attending genetic counselling for familial breast or ovarian cancer: a questionnaire, interview, and observational study', *British Medical Journal*, 314 (7076): 281.

Hallowell, N., Arden-Jones, A., Eeles, R., Foster, C., Lucassen, A., Moynihan, C. and Watson, M. (2006) 'Guilt, blame and responsibility: men's understanding of their role in the transmission of BRCA1/2 mutations within their family', *Sociology of Health & Illness*, 28 (7): 969–88.

Hamel, N., Feng, B.J., Foretova, L., Stoppa-Lyonnet, D., Narod, S.A., Imyanitov, E., Sinilnikova, O., Tihomirova, L., Lubinski, J., Gronwald, J., Gorski, B., Hansen, T., Nielsen, F.C., Thomassen, M., Yannoukakos, D., Konstantopoulou, I., Zajac, V., Ciernikova, S., Couch, F.J., Greenwood, C.M.T., Goldgar, D.E. and Foulkes, W.D. (2011) 'On the origin and diffusion of BRCA1 c.5266dupC (5382insC) in European populations', *European Journal of Human Genetics*, 19 (3): 300–6.

HapMap Project (2011) 'How Are Ethical Issues Being Addressed?' Online, http://snp.cshl.org/ethicalconcerns.html.en (accessed 13 January 2012).

Hashiloni-Dolev, Y. (2006) 'Between mothers, fetuses and society: reproductive genetics in the Israeli-Jewish context', *Nashim: A Journal of Jewish Women's Studies & Gender Issues*, 12 (1): 129–50.

JACOB (Jews against Cancer of the Breast) (2011) Online, http://www.jacobintl.org/ (accessed 22 December 2011).

Jasanoff, S. (ed.) (2004) *States of Knowledge: The Co-production of Science and Social Order*, London: Routledge.

Kaback, M.M. (2000) 'Population-based genetic screening for reproductive counseling: the Tay-Sachs disease model', *European Journal of Pediatrics*, 159 (15): 192–5.

Kahn, S.M. (2000) *Reproducing Jews: A Cultural Account of Assisted Conception in Israel*, Durham, NC: Duke University Press.

Kahn, S.M. (2005) 'Are genes Jewish? Conceptual ambiguities in the new genetic age'. Paper presented at Jean and Samuel Center for Judaic Studies, University of Michigan, 16 March 2005.

Kenen, R. (1996) 'The at-risk health status and technology: a diagnostic invitation and the "gift" of knowing', *Social Science and Medicine*, 42 (22): 1545–53.

Kirsh, N. (2003) 'Population genetics in Israel in the 1950s', *Isis*, 94 (4): 631–55.

Kronn, D., Jansen, V. and Ostrer, H. (1998) 'Carrier screening for cystic fibrosis, Gaucher disease, and Tay-Sachs disease in the Ashkenazi Jewish population: the First 1000 cases at New York University Medical Center, New York, NY', *Archives of Internal Medicine*, 158 (7): 777–81.

Latour, B. and Woolgar, S. (1979) *Laboratory Life: The Social Construction of Scientific Facts*, London: Sage.

Lawton, J., Ahmard, N., Peel, E. and Hallowell, N. (2007) 'Contextualising accounts of illness: notions of responsibility and blame in white South Asian respondents' accounts of diabetes causation', *Sociology of Health & Illness*, 29 (6): 891–906.

Lehman, L.S., Weeks, J.C., Klar, N. and Garber, J. (2002) 'A population based study of Ashkenazi Jewish women's attitudes toward genetic discrimination and BRCA1/2 testing', *Genetics in Medicine*, 4 (5): 346–52.

Lerman, C., Narod, S., Schulman, K., Hughes, C., Gomez-Caminero, A., Bonney, G., Gold, K., Trock, B., Main, D., Lynch, J., Fulmore, C., Snyder, C., Lemon, S.J., Conway, T., Tonin, P., Lenoir, G. and Lynch, H. (1996) 'BRCA1 testing in families with hereditary breast–ovarian cancer: a prospective study of patient decision making and outcomes', *Journal of the American Medical Association*, 275 (24): 1885–92.

Levene, S. (2005) 'Genetic screening in the Ashkenazi Jewish population – is there a case for more testing?', Report for the National Screening Committee on the meeting held on 3 June 2004 at Guy's Hospital, London.

Levin, M. (2003) 'Ethical, cultural and religious aspects of hereditary cancer in Jewish communities', *Cancer Therapy*, 1: 269–73.

Levy-Lahad, E., Catane, R., Eisenberg, S., Kaufman, B., Hornreich, G., Lishinsky E., Shohat, M., Weber, B.L., Beller, U., Lahad, A. and Halle, D. (1997) 'Founder BRCA1 and BRCA2 mutations in Ashkenazi Jews in Israel: frequency and differential penetrance in ovarian cancer and in breast–ovarian cancer families', *American Journal of Human Genetics*, 60 (5): 1059–67.

Levy-Lahad, E., Gabai-Kapara, E., Kaufman, B., Catane, C., Regev, S., Renbaum, P., Beller, U., King, M.-C. and Lahad, A. (2011) 'Evidence for population-based screening of BRCA1 and BRCA' (program number 1191T). Presented at the 12th International Congress of Human Genetics/61st Annual Meeting of the American Society of Human Genetics, 13 October 2011, Montreal, Canada.

Lock, M. (1998) 'Breast cancer: reading the omens', *Anthropology Today*, 14 (4): 7–16.

Lodder, L.N., Frets, P.G., Trijsburg, R.W., Meijers-Heijboer, E.J., Klijn, J.G.M., Duivenvoorden, H.J., Tibben, A., Wagner, A., van der Meer, C.A., Devilee, P., Cornelisse, C.J. and Niermeijer, M.F. (1999) 'Presymptomatic testing for BRCA1 and BRCA2: how distressing are the pre-test weeks?', *Journal of Medical Genetics*, 36 (12): 906–13.

Lodder L.N., Frets, P.G., Trijsburg, R.W., Meijers-Heijboer, E.J., Klijn, J.G.M., Duivenvoorden, H.J., Tibben, A., Wagner, A., van der Meer, C.A., van den Ouweland, A.M.W. and Niermeijer, M.F. (2001) 'Psychological impact of receiving a BRCA1/ BRCA2 test result', *American Journal of Medical Genetics*, 98 (1): 15–24.

London Jewish Cultural Centre (2007) 'Intermarriage – was it ever a good thing?', course offered in May 2007.

Lowy, I. and Gaudilliere, J.P. (2008) 'Localizing the global: testing for hereditary risks of breast cancer', *Science, Technology & Human Values*, 33: 299–325.

Luna, F. (2009) 'Elucidating the concept of vulnerability: layers not labels', *International Journal of Feminist Approaches to Bioethics*, 2 (1): 121–39.

Lyall, S. (2009) 'Who is a Jew? Court ruling in Britain raises questions', *New York Times*, 8 September 2009. Online, http://www.nytimes.com/2009/11/08/world/europe/08britain.html?pagewanted=all (accessed 22 December 2011).

Lynch, H.T., Lemon, S.J. and Durham, C. (1997) 'A descriptive study of BRCA 1 testing and reactions to disclosure of test results', *Cancer*, 79: 2219–28.

Markel, H. (1997) 'Di Goldine Medina (the golden land): historical perspectives of eugenics and the East European (Ashkenazi) Jewish American community, 1880–1925', *Health Matrix: Journal of Law-Medicine*, 7 (1): 49–64.

Marks, J. (2002) 'Genes, bodies and species', pp. 14–28 in P. Peregrine and M. Ember (eds) *Physical Anthropology: Original Readings in Method and Practice*, Upper Saddle River, NJ: Prentice Hall.

Marks, J. (2008) 'Race: past, present and future', pp. 21–38 in B. Koenig, S.-J. Lee and S. Richardson (eds) *Revisiting Race in a Genomic Age*, New Brunswick, NJ: Rutgers University Press.

Marshall, G. (1993) 'Racial Classification: Popular and Scientific', pp. 116–27 in S. Harding (ed.) *The 'Racial' Economy of Science*, Bloomington, IN: Indiana University Press.

Martin, E. (1998) 'Anthropology and the cultural study of science', *Science, Technology & Human Values*, 23 (1): 24–44.

M'Charek, A. (2005) *The Human Genome Diversity Project: An Ethnography of Scientific Practise*, Cambridge: Cambridge University Press.

Metcalfe, K.A., Poll, A., Royer, R., Llacuachaqui, M., Tulman, A., Sun, P. and Narod, S.A. (2009) 'Screening for founder mutations in BRCA1 and BRCA2 in unselected Jewish women', *Journal of Clinical Oncology*, 28: 387–91.

Michael, M. and Birke, L. (1994) 'Accounting for animal experiments: identity and disreputable "others"', *Science, Technology & Human Values*, 19 (2): 189–204.

Michie, S., Bobrow, M. and Marteau, T.M. (2001) 'Predictive genetic testing in children and adults: a study of emotional impact', *Journal of Medical Genetics*, 38 (8): 519–26.

Miki, Y., Swensen, J., Shattuck-Eidens, D., Futreal, PA., Harshman, K., Tavtigian, S., Liu, Q., Cochran, C., Bennett, L.M. and Ding, W. (1994) 'A strong candidate for the breast and ovarian cancer susceptibility gene BRCA1', *Science*, 266 (5182): 66–71.

Modell, B. and Darr, A. (2002) 'Genetic counselling and customary consanguineous marriage', *Nature Review Genetics*, 3 (3): 225–9.

Montoya, M.J. (2007) 'Bioethnic conscription: genes, race, and Mexicana/o ethnicity in diabetes research', *Cultural Anthropology*, 22 (1): 94–128.

Mor, P. and Oberle, K. (2008) 'Ethical issues related to BRCA gene testing in Orthodox Jewish women', *Nursing Ethics*, 15 (4): 512–22.

Motulsky, A.G. and Fraser, G.R. (1980) 'Effects of antenatal diagnosis and selective abortion on frequencies of genetic disorders', *Clinics in Obstetrics and Gynaecology*, 7 (1): 121–33.

Movement for Reform Judaism UK (2011) 'Abortion'. Online, http://www.reformjudaism.org.uk/a-to-z-of-reform-judaism/medical-ethics/abortion.html (accessed 22 December 2011).

Mozersky, J. and Joseph, G. (2010) 'Case studies in the co-production of populations and genetics: the making of "at risk" populations in BRCA genetics', *Biosocieties*, 5 (4): 415–39.

Murray, C. (2007) 'Jewish genius', *Commentary Magazine*. Online, http://www.commentarymagazine.com/article/jewish-genius/ (accessed 13 January 2012).

Narod, S. (2009) 'Screening for BRCA1 and BRCA2 mutations in breast cancer patients from Mexico: the public health perspective', *Salud Publica de Mexico*, 51d (2): S191–6.

National Cancer Institute (1995) 'Scientists report new lead in the genetics of breast cancer', 28 September 1995. Online, http://archive.hhs.gov/news/press/1995pres/950928a.html (accessed 22 December 2011).

National Cancer Institute (2011) 'Genetics of breast and ovarian cancer physician data query'. Online, http://www.cancer.gov/cancertopics/pdq/genetics/breast-and-ovarian/HealthProfessional (accessed 22 December 2011).

National Institute of Clinical Excellence (NICE) (2005) 'Familial breast cancer: full guideline'. Online, http://guidance.nice.org.uk/CG41/Guidance/pdf/English (accessed 13 January 2012).

Nelson, A. (2008) 'Bio science: genetic genealogy testing and the pursuit of African ancestry', *Social Studies of Science*, 38 (5): 759–83.

Nelson, H.D., Huffman, L.H., Fu, R. and Harris, E.L. (2005) 'Genetic risk assessment and BRCA mutation testing for breast and ovarian cancer susceptibility: systematic evidence review for the U.S. Preventive Services Task Force', *Annals of Internal Medicine*, 43 (5): 362–79.

Neuhausen, S.L., Godwin, A.K., Gershoni-Baruch, R., Schubert, E., Garber, J., Stoppa-Lyonnet, D., Olah, E., Csokay, B., Serova, O., Lalloo, F., Osorio, A., Stratton, M., Offit, K., Boyd, J., Caligo, M.A., Scott, R.J., Schofield, A., Teugels, E., Schwab, M., Cannon-Albright, L., Bishop, T., Easton, D., Benitez, J., King, M.C., Ponder, B.A.J., Weber, B., Devilee, P., Borg, Å., Narod, S.A. and Goldgar, D. (1998) 'Haplotype and phenotype analysis of nine recurrent BRCA2 mutations in 111 families: results of an international study', *American Journal of Human Genetics*, 62 (6): 1381–8.

Neulander, J.S. (2006) 'Folk taxonomy, prejudice and the human genome: using disease as a Jewish ethnic marker', *Patterns of Prejudice*, 40: 381–98.

Novas, C. and Rose, N. (2000) 'Genetic risk and the birth of the somatic individual', *Economy and Society*, 29: 485–513.

Obasogie, O.K. (2009) 'Playing the gene card? A report on race and human biotechnology', *Center for Genetics and Society*. Online, http://www.geneticsandsociety.org/article.php?id=4465 (accessed 12 January 2012).

Oller, D.T. (1984) 'Jewish genetic diseases and Jewish illness behavior: a review of selected sociocultural literature', *Jewish Social Studies*, 46 (2): 177–87.

Olopade, O.F. (2004) 'Genetics in clinical cancer care: a promise unfulfilled among minority populations', *Cancer Epidemiology, Biomarkers & Prevention*, 13 (11): 1683–6.

Olopade, O.F., Williams, C.K. and Falkson, C.I. (eds) (2005) *Breast Cancer in Women of African Descent*, Netherlands: Springer.

Ossorio, P. and Duster, T. (2005) 'Race and genetics: controversies in biomedical, behavioural and forensic science', *American Psychologist*, 60 (1): 115–28.

Parthasarathy, S. (2007) *Building Genetic Medicine: Breast Cancer, Technology, and the Comparative Politics of Health Care*, Cambridge, MA: MIT Press.

Petersen, A. (2003) 'Governmentality, critical scholarship, and the medical humanities', *Journal of Medical Humanities*, 24 (3): 187–201.

Phillips, K.A., Warner, E., Meschino, W.S., Hunter, J., Abdolell, M., Glendon, G., Andrulis, I.L. and Goodwin, P.J. (2000) 'Perceptions of Ashkenazi Jewish breast cancer patients on genetic testing for mutations in BRCA1 and BRCA2', *Clinical Genetics*, 57 (5): 376–83.

Prainsack, B. (2006) '"Negotiating life"': the regulation of human cloning and embryonic stem cell research in Israel', *Social Studies of Science*, 36: 173–205.

Prainsack, B. (2007) 'Research populations: biobanks in Israel', *New Genetics & Society*, 26: 85–103.

Prainsack, B. and Firestine, O. (2006) 'Science for survival: biotechnology regulation in Israel', *Science & Public Policy*, 33: 33–46.

Prainsack, B. and Siegal, G. (2006) 'The rise of genetic couplehood? A comparative view of premarital genetic testing', *Biosocieties*, 1 (1): 17–36.

Press, N., Burke, W. and Durfy, S.J. (1997) 'How are Jewish women different from all other women? Anthropological perspectives on genetic susceptibility testing for breast cancer', *Health Matrix: Journal of Law-Medicine*, 7: 135–62.

Priest, L. (2008) 'Cancer test a genetic crystal ball for women', *Globe and Mail*, 24 May 2008. Online, http://www.theglobeandmail.com/life/cancer-test-a-genetic-crystal-ball-for-jewish-women/article687467/ (accessed 22 December 2011).

Proctor, R. (1999) *The Nazi War on Cancer*, Princeton, NJ: Princeton University Press.

Rabinovitch, D. (2007) *Take off Your Party Dress: When Life's Too Busy for Breast Cancer*, London: Simon & Schuster.

Rabinow, P. (1996) 'Artificiality and enlightenment: from sociobiology to biosociality', pp. 91–111 in P. Rabinow, *Essays on the Anthropology of Reason*, Princeton, NJ: Princeton University Press.

Rapp, R. (2000) *Testing Women, Testing the Fetus*, New York: Routledge.

Raz, A.E. (2010) *Community Genetics and Genetic Alliances: Eugenics, Carrier Testing and Networks of Risk*, Abingdon: Routledge.

Reardon, J. (2005) *'Race to the Finish' Identity and Governance in un Age of Genomics*, Princeton, NJ: Princeton University Press.

Reardon, J. (2007) 'Democratic mishaps: the problem of democratization in a time of biopolitics', *Biosocieties*, 2: 239–56.

Report of the Anglo-Israeli workshop on the genetic risk of breast cancer (2006), unpublished report of meeting held in Israel 22–6 April 2006.

Richards, M. (1996) 'Families, kinship and genetics', pp. 249–73 in T.M. Marteau and M. Richards (eds) *The Troubled Helix: Social and Psychological Implications of the New Human Genetics*, Cambridge: Cambridge University Press.

Risch, N., Burchard, E., Ziv, E. and Tang, H. (2002) 'Categorization of humans in biomedical research: genes, race and disease', *Genome Biology*, 3 (7): comment.

Risch, N., de Leon, D., Ozelius, L., Kramer, P., Almasy, L., Singer, B., Fahn, S., Breakefield, X. and Bressman, S. (1995) 'Genetic analysis of idiopathic torsion dystonia in Ashkenazi Jews and their recent descent from a small founder population', *Nature Genetics*, 9 (2): 152–9.

Risch, N., Tang, H., Katzenstein, H. and Ekstein, J. (2003) 'Geographic distribution of disease mutations in the Ashkenazi Jewish population supports genetic drift over selection', *American Journal of Human Genetics*, 72 (4): 812–22.

Robson, M.E., Storm, C.D., Weitzel, J., Wollins, D.S. and Offit, K. (2010) 'American Society of Clinical Oncology policy statement update: genetic and genomic testing for cancer susceptibility', *Journal of Clinical Oncology*, 28 (5): 893–901.

Rose, N. (2007) *Politics of Life Itself: Biomedicine, Power and Subjectivity in the Twenty-First Century*, Princeton, NJ: Princeton University Press.

Rosner, F. (2001) *Biomedical Ethics and Jewish Law*, Hoboken, NJ: KTAV Publishing House.

Rothenberg, K. (1997) 'Breast cancer, the genetic "quick fix" and the Jewish community', *Health Matrix: Journal of Law-Medicine*, 7 (1): 97–124.

Rothenberg, K. (2000) 'Report of the first community consultation on the responsible collection and use of samples for genetic research for the National Institute of General Medical Sciences', National Institute of the General Medical Sciences. Online, http://www.nigms.nih.gov/News/Reports/community_consultation.htm (accessed 22 December 2011).

Schwartz, M.D., Peshkin, B.N., Hughes, C., Main, D., Isaacs, C. and Lerman, C. (2002) 'Impact of BRCA1/BRCA2 mutation testing on psychologic distress in a clinic-based sample', *Journal of Clinical Oncology*, 20 (2): 514–20.

Seale, C. (2004) *Researching Society and Culture*, London: Sage.

Sharsheret: Your Jewish Community Facing Breast Cancer (2011). Online, http://www. sharsheret.org/ (accessed 22 December 2011).

Shkedi-Rafid, S. (2012) 'Screening for susceptibility genes: the point of view of asymptomatic carriers with no family history of the tested condition; and attitudes of health-care providers toward population screening', unpublished PhD thesis. To be submitted to the Hebrew University of Jerusalem.

Skinner, D. (2007) 'Groundhog day? The strange case of sociology, race and "science"', *Sociology*, 41 (5): 931–43.

Slatkin, M. (2004) 'A population-genetic test of founder effects and implications for Ashkenazi Jewish diseases', *American Journal of Human Genetics*, 75: 282–93.

Sontag, S. (1990) *Illness as Metaphor; and AIDS and Its Metaphor*, New York: Random House.

Stolberg, S.G. (1998) 'Concern among Jews is heightened as scientists deepen genetic studies', *New York Times*, 22 April 1998.

Stone, L., Lurquin, P.F. and Cavalli-Sforza, L.L. (2007) *Genes, Culture and Human Evolution: A Synthesis*, Oxford: Blackwell Publishing.

Strathern, M. (1992) *Reproducing the Future: Anthropology, Kinship and the New Reproductive Technologies*, New York: Routledge.

Struewing, J.P., Hartge, P., Wacholder, S., Baker, S.M., Berlin, M., McAdams, M., Timmerman, M.M., Brody, L.C. and Tucker, M.A. (1997) 'The risk of cancer associated with specific mutations of BRCA1 and BRCA2 among Ashkenazi Jews', *New England Journal of Medicine*, 336 (20): 1401–8.

Symons, L. (2006) 'Cancer breakthrough', *Jewish Chronicle*, 5 May 2006: 2.

Taussig, K.S., Rapp, R. and Heath, D. (2003) 'Flexible eugenics: technologies of the self in the age of genetics', pp.58–76 in A.H. Goodman, D. Heath and M.S. Lindee (eds) *Genetic Nature/Culture: Anthropology and Science beyond the Two-Culture Divide*, Berkeley, CA: University of California Press.

Tate, S.K. and Goldstein, D.B. (2004) 'Will tomorrow's medicines work for everyone?', *Nature Genetics*, 36: S34–S42.

Thomas, M.G., Parfitt, T., Weiss, D.A., Skorecki, K., Wilson, J.F., le Roux, M., Bradman, N. and Goldstein, D.B.Y (2000) 'Chromosomes traveling south: the Cohen modal haplotype and the origins of the Lemba, the black Jews of Southern Africa', *American Journal of Human Genetics*, 66 (2): 674–86.

United Nations Educational, Scientific and Cultural Organisation (UNESCO) (1950) 'The race question'. Online, http://unesdoc.unesco.org/images/0012/001282/128291eo.pdf (accessed 22 December 2011).

United Synagogue of Conservative Judaism (1999) 'Genetic testing, discrimination and the Jewish community 1999 resolution by the United Synagogue'. Online, http://uscj2004.aptinet.com/Genetic_Testing_Disc6690.html (accessed 22 December 2011).

Wailoo, K. and Pemberton, S. (2006) *The Troubled Dream of Genetic Medicine: Ethnicity and Innovation in Tay Sachs, Cystic Fibrosis and Sickle Cell Disease*, Baltimore, MD: Johns Hopkins University Press.

Watson, M., Foster, C., Eeles, R., Eccles, D., Ashley, S., Davidson, R., Mackay, J., Morrison, P.J., Hopwood, P. and Evans, D.G.R. (2004) 'Psychosocial impact of breast/ovarian (BRCA 1/2) cancer-predictive genetic testing in a UK multi-centre clinical cohort', *British Journal of Cancer*, 91 (10): 1787–94.

Watson, M., Lloyd, S.M. and Eeles, R. (1996) 'Psychosocial impact of testing (by linkage) for the BRCA1 breast cancer gene: an investigation of two families in the research setting', *Psycho-Oncology*, 5: 233–9.

Weiler, J.H.H. (2010) 'Discrimination and identity in London', *Jewish Review of Books*, No. 1, Spring 2010. Online, http://www.jewishreviewofbooks.com/publications/detail/discrimination-and-identity-in-london-the-jewish-free-school-case (accessed 22 December 2011).

Weitzel, J.N., Lagos, V.I., Blazer, K.R., Nelson, R., Ricker, C., Herzog, J., McGuire, C. and Neuhausen, S. (2005) 'Prevalence of BRCA mutations and founder effect in high-risk Hispanic families', *Cancer Epidemiology, Biomarkers & Prevention*, 14 (7): 1666–71.

Weitzel, J.N., Lagos, V.I., Herzog, J.S., Judkins, T., Hendrickson, B., Ho, J.S., Ricker, C.N., Lowstuter, K.J., Blazer, K.R., Tomlinson, G. and Scholl, T. (2007) 'Evidence for common ancestral origin of a recurring BRCA1 genomic rearrangement identified in high-risk Hispanic families', *Cancer Epidemiology, Biomarkers & Prevention*, 16 (8): 1615–20.

White House (2000) 'President Clinton announces the completion of the first draft of the human genome', Office of the Press Secretary. Online, http://www.ornl.gov/sci/techresources/Human_Genome/project/clinton1.shtml (accessed 22 December 2011).

Wooster, R., Bignell, G., Lancaster, J., Swift, S., Seal, S., Mangion, J., Collins, N., Gregory, S., Gumbs, C. and Micklem, G. (1995) 'Identification of the breast cancer susceptibility gene BRCA2', *Nature*, 378 (6559): 789–92.

Zavestoski, S., McCormick, S. and Brown, P. (2004) 'Gender, embodiment, and disease: environmental breast cancer activists' challenges to science, the biomedical model, and policy', *Science as Culture*, 13 (4): 563–86.

Zertal, I. (2000) 'From the People's Hall to the Wailing Wall: a study in memory, fear, and war', *Representations*, 69: 96–126.

Ziogas, D.E., Christos, S.K. and Roukos, D.H. (2011) 'Preventing familial breast and ovarian cancer: major research advances with little implication', *Women's Health*, 7 (2): 135–8.

Index